Medicines and Risk/Benefit Decisions

CMR Workshop Series

Monitoring for Adverse Drug Reactions
Editors: S.R. Walker and A. Goldberg

Long-Term Animal Studies
Their Predictive Value for Man
Editors: S.R. Walker and A.D. Dayan

Medicines and Risk/Benefit Decisions
Editors: S.R. Walker and A.W. Asscher

Quality of Life – Assessment and Application
Editor: S.R. Walker

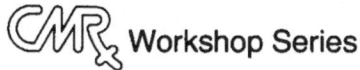 Workshop Series

Medicines and Risk/Benefit Decisions

EDITED BY

Stuart R Walker

Director of the Centre for Medicines Research
Carshalton, Surrey

and

A William Asscher

Professor of Renal Medicine
University of Wales College of Medicine
Royal Infirmary, Cardiff

*Proceedings of Centre for Medicines Research Workshop
held at the Ciba Foundation, London
October 1, 1985*

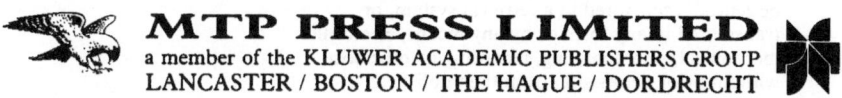

MTP PRESS LIMITED
a member of the KLUWER ACADEMIC PUBLISHERS GROUP
LANCASTER / BOSTON / THE HAGUE / DORDRECHT

Published in the UK and Europe by
MTP Press Limited
Falcon House
Lancaster, England

British Library Cataloguing in Publication Data

Medicines and risk/benefit decisions : proceedings of
   Centre for Medicines Research Workshop held at the
   Ciba Foundation, London, October 1, 1985. — (CMR workshop series)
   1. Drugs—Safety measures   2. Drugs—Testing
   I. Walker, Stuart R.   II. Asscher, A.W.
   III. Series
   363.1'9475   RM301

Published in the USA by
MTP Press
A division of Kluwer Boston Inc
101 Philip Drive
Norwell, MA 02061, USA

Library of Congress Cataloging-in-Publication Data

Centre for Medicines Research (Surrey). Workshop
   (1985 : Ciba Foundation)
   Medicines and risk/benefit decisions.

   (CMR workshop series)
   "Proceeding of Centre for Medicines Research
   Workshop held at the Ciba Foundation, London,
   October 1, 1985."
   Includes bibliographies and index.
   1. Drugs—Effectiveness—Congresses.   2. Drugs—
   Toxicology—Congresses.   3. Chemotherapy—
   Decision making—Congresses.   I. Walker, Stuart
   R., 1944-   .   II. Asscher, A.W.   III. Title.
   IV. Series.   [DNLM: 1. Decision Making—congresses.
   2. Medicine—congresses.   3. Probability—congresses.
   4. Research—congresses.   W 20.5 C397m 1985]
   RM301.C44   1985   615.5'8   86–27267

   ISBN 978-94-010-7946-4   ISBN 978-94-009-3221-0 (eBook)
   DOI 10.1007/978-94-009-3221-0

Phototypeset by Witwell Ltd, Liverpool, England.

Contents

Preface

The third CMR Workshop provided the opportunity for a group of experts from the Industry, academia and the regulatory authorities to meet and discuss ways and means by which risk benefit decisions are made during the various stages of drug development. It became apparent from the discussions that took place in October 1985, at the CIBA Foundation, that decisions are often made with limited data and inadequate methodology. The conclusions drawn from the day's deliberations were as follows:

1. Current methodology for assessing risk and particularly benefits must be improved;
2. Safety must be assessed in association with benefits as it is ultimately the benefit/risk ratio which should decide the future of medicines;
3. Risks from medicines must always be viewed in relation to the risks from untreated diseases.

It seemed to be the consensus of the group that such a meeting was both useful and informative and, hopefully, the publication of these proceedings will stimulate further discussion in this important area which may improve the decision-making process in drug development.

The Editors wish to thank the participants for contributing to the Workshop, together with Dr. Cyndy Lumley for providing the initial transcript of the meeting and Mrs Sheila Wright for producing the final version and for carrying out all the additional work that is entailed in producing such a publication.

Professor S. R. Walker
Professor A. W. Asscher

Foreword

Professor R Hurley

Since the licensing of medicinal products is based on risk/benefit decisions it is essential that the nature, both of risk and benefit, should be addressed closely, as was attempted in the Centre for Medicines Research Workshop, the proceedings of which are published here.

Most speakers concurred that the perception of risk and, more importantly, its acceptability are highly individual, emphasising the central dilemma of regulatory authorities who must take decisions based on data that pertain to groups. Crucial, however, is the requirement to communicate, in the fullest form, data on risk to doctors, patients and public, and to educate them to the understanding that risk/benefit analysis is a dynamic process. This starts with decisions taken early in a drug's development, progressing through those of the investigational and licensing stages and continues in the post-marketing phase.

The assessment of benefit is no less problematical than that of risk, for here too value judgements must operate; freedom from particular types of morbidity may be more desired than postponement of death, hampering the interpretation of clinical data. Some economic benefits are demonstrable but those pertinent to psychosocial well-being are elusive. The concept of quality of life has gained credence in the last twenty years and beliefs about health need to be explored more thoroughly. In some circumstances, measures derived from study of the individual as the unit may be applicable to a group.

In reaching decisions on licensing the United Kingdom Authority and its expert committees are bound by the Medicines Act to consider efficacy, safety and quality. Once a drug is licensed, it is the practitioner who must interpret the risk/benefit equation for individual patients. Licensed medicines are subject to review and as data accumulates, the risk/benefit ratio may shift and medicines may be withdrawn. Even in these circumstances, evidence of efficacy may be uncertain, hazards may be incompletely defined and risk difficult to quantitate.

The Workshop focussed on the many deficiences in the data on which risk/benefit decisions have to be made. Suggestions for extension and refinement of the database were made. Improvement in post-marketing surveillance is seen by many as cardinal in this development.

Notes on Contributors

Dame Elizabeth Ackroyd, is Chairman of the Patients' Association.

Professor A. W. Asscher, BSc, MD, FRCP, is Professsor of Renal Medicine at the University of Wales College of Medicine in Cardiff. His research interests are in the field of urinary tract infections. He has served on the Medicines Commission, and is at present Chairman of the Committee on the Review of Medicines and Chairman-elect of the Committee on the Safety of Medicines.

Professor R. Bass, MD, was Postdoctoral Fellow with Professor A.L. Lehninger at The John Hopkins School of Medicine, Department of Physiological Chemistry, Baltimore, USA and Postdoctoral Fellow and Assistant Professor of Pharmacology with Professor Neubert at the Free University, Institute of Toxicology and Embryopharmakologie, Berlin. From 1979 he was Head of Toxicology and Director and Professor at the Institute for Drugs of the Federal Health Office Berlin and since 1984 Auberplanmabiger Professor of Pharmacology and Toxicology at the Free University, Berlin. Todays research interests are in reproduction and short-term tests in toxicology. He has had over 90 papers, articles and books published in this area on formaldehyde, animal experiments and protection and regulatory toxicology.

Dr. R.W. Brimblecombe, MSc, PhD, DSc, FRCPath, is Vice President, Research and Development, at Smith, Kline and French Laboratories. He leads the UK-based R&D groups sited at The Frythe near Welwyn in Hertfordshire and at Tonbridge in Kent. He also has overall responsibility for Smith Kline & French R&D related activities in Japan. He is the author of three books and about 100 other publications mainly in the fields of endocrinology, neuropharmacology, toxicology and drug development.

Dr B.W. Cromie, MB, FRCP(Ed), is currently Director of Hoechst UK Ltd, Chairman of Pharmaceutical Division, Chairman of Arthur H. Cox and Co. Ltd, Member of the Board of Management of the ABPI, Fellow of Green College, Oxford, and is also a Member of the Institute of Medical Ethics Working Party. Recent past appointments include Commissioner of Medicines Commission, Member of Home Office Advisory Committee on Animal Experimentation and Member of the Code of Practice Committee of ABPI.

Professor C.T. Dollery, BSc, MB, ChB, FRCP, has research interests which are almost entirely concerned with the actions of drugs upon the regulation of the cardio-pulmonary system and are currently expressed in two main projects. One is concerned with the regulation of the sympathetic nervous system with special reference to blood pressure control, and the second in the products of arachidonic acid metabolism and their role in the lung in asthma and in the blood vessels in vascular disease.

Dr J.D. Fitzgerald, MB, BSc, FRCP, is currently International Medical Director of the Pharmaceuticals Division of ICI plc. He has been involved in drug discovery and development for twenty years, having been responsible for the human evaluation of gastrointestinal, metabolic and cardiovascular drugs. He has also had experience in teaching therapeutics whilst Professor of Pharmacology at McMaster University, Hamilton, Ontario, Canada as well as directing pre-clinical research in a range of therapeutic fields.

Professor C.F. George, BSc, MD, FRCP, is Professor of Clinical Pharmacology and Deputy Dean of the Faculty of Medicine, University of Southampton. He is Secretary to the Editorial Board of the *British Journal of Clinical Pharmacology*, and is a member of the Committee on the Review of Medicines and the Administration of Radioactive Substances Advisory Committee. His research interests include cardiovascular clinical pharmacology, pre-systemic drug metabolism and the use of prescription information leaflets.

Professor Sir A. Goldberg, MD, DSc, FRCP, FRS(Ed), is Regius Professor of the Practice of Medicine at the University of Glasgow and Chairman of the Committee on Safety of Medicines. He has been involved in research of blood diseases and clinical pharmacology and disorders of porphyrin metabolism. He is Chairman of the Examining Board for the Diploma in Pharmaceutical Medicine and has been active in the encouragement of this discipline.

Professor Rosalinde Hurley, LLB, MD, FRCPath, is Professor of Microbiology at the Institute of Obstetrics and Gynaecology, now part of the Royal Postgraduate Medical School. Her research interests include fungal diseases, in particular the mycoses associated with *Candida* species, infections of the central nervous system (brain abscess and neonatal meningitis), and virus infections during pregnancy. She was formerly Chairman of the Committee on Dental and Surgical Materials, and has been Chairman of the Medicines Commission since 1982. Formerly a member of the Board of Governors of Queen Charlotte's Hospital for Women, she is a member of the Public Health Laboratory Service Board and is Chairman of the District Medical Advisory Committee and a member of the District Management Board of Hammersmith and Queen Charlotte's Special Health Authority. She is an Honorary Secretary of the Royal Society of Medicine.

Dr D. Irvine, OBE, is a principal in general practice in Ashington, Northumberland and Regional Adviser in General Practice in the University of Newcastle. Immediate past Chairman, Council of the Royal College of General Practitioners, he is presently a Member of the GMC and Chairman of its Standards Committee. His research interests include quality assurance through the Northern Region Study of Standards and Performance Review in General Practice.

Dr C.R.B. Joyce, PhD, FBPsS, is Head of Project Innovation in the Ciba–Geigy (Basle) Medical Department, and is an Associate of the University of Colorado at Boulder, USA. His main research interests are the development of patient-oriented methods and the study of clinical and managerial judgment.

Professor D.H. Lawson, MD, FRCP(Ed), is Consultant Physician at Glasgow Royal Infirmary, Visiting Professor in the School of Pharmaceutical Sciences at the University of Strathclyde and Visiting Consultant at the Boston Collaborative Drug Surveillance Program, Boston University. He has been a member of the Committee on the Review of Medicines since 1979 and its Vice

Chairman since 1985. His research interests relate primarily to the epidemiology of adverse drug reactions.

Professor T.R. Lee, MA, PhD, FBPsS, has, as his main research interest, environmental psychology, but he has also conducted research in industry, education and other fields of applied psychology. At present he leads a research group concerned with risk perception and public attitudes to nuclear power stations, radioactive waste management facilities and other environmental hazards.

Professor M.D. Rawlins, BSc, MD, FRCP, is Professor of Clinical Pharmacology at the University of Newcastle upon Tyne and Consultant Clinical Pharmacologist to the Newcastle Health Authority. He is a member of the Committee on the Safety of Medicines, the subcommittee on Safety, Efficacy and Adverse Reactions (SEAR) and Chairman of its Adverse Reactions Group (ARGOS). Professor Rawlins' research interests are primarily concerned with elucidating sources of variability in response to drugs, mechanisms of adverse drug reactions and in monitoring their usage and effects.

Professor A. Smith, PhD, FRCP, FFCM, FRCGP, is Professor of Epidemiology and Social Oncology in Manchester, and is Head of a department engaged in research designed to provide a rational basis for and a continuous appraisal of a regional strategy for cancer control concerned with the organization of the prevention, early detection and treatment of cancer and the care of cancer patients.

Professor G. Teeling Smith, OBE, BA, FPS, HonMPharm, has been Director of the Office of Health Economics since its foundation in 1962. His special areas of interest are the economics of pharmaceutical innovation and the measurement of the social and economic benefits which result from improvements in therapy. His research also covers the organization and benefits of health care generally, both in Britain and in other countries. Since 1970 he has been teaching undergraduate and postgraduate students in health economics at Brunel University.

Dr J. Urquhart, MD, is co-founder and President of APREX Corporation which makes compliance-monitoring/facilitating pharmaceutical packaging. With Professor Klaus Heilmann and H.A.J. Struyker-Boudier he is the co-author of RISK WATCH and its German and Dutch versions, which defines the Safety-degree Scale for facilitating public communication of technology- and drug-related risk. He is also Adjunct Professor of Pharmacy at the University of California Medical Center, San Francisco, Visiting Professor of Pharmaco-epidemiology at the University of Limburg, Maastricht, Netherlands and serves on the Advisory Committee to the Director of the US National Institutes of Health.

Professor D.W. Vere, MD, FRCP, holds a Chair in Therapeutics at the London Hospital Medical College, London. He is Director of the Department of Pharmacology and Therapeutics at the College and Consultant Physician to the London Hospital. His research work includes the design of clinical trials, drug strategies in pain relief and methods to study compliance with treatment.

Professor S.R. Walker, BSc, PhD, CChem, FRSC, is Director of the Centre for Medicines Research and Honorary Professor of the Welsh School of Pharmacy, Cardiff. His current research involves an assessment of the innovation and development of new medicines, investigating the predictive value of pre-clinical animal toxicology, and determining ways of assessing the burden of adverse drug reactions in primary care and improving the methodology for voluntary reporting. He is the author of over 100 research papers and four books.

Professor G. Zbinden, MD, FRCPath, was trained in pathology and paediatrics and worked for the drug company Hoffmann-la Roche and Co. AG, first as Head of Toxicology in Basle, Switzerland and then as Director of Research in Nutley, New Jersey, USA. He then spent 3 years at the Department of Medicine of the University of Cambridge, England and became Professor of Experimental Pathology and later Professor of Toxicology at the University of Zurich, Switzerland. He is now Director of the Institute of Toxicology of the Swiss Federal Institute of Technology and the University of Zurich in Schwerzenbach, Switzerland. His interests are mainly toxicological model systems for the evaluation of safety of drugs and other chemicals.

Introductory remarks

Professor S. R. Walker

Obviously it is not my duty to anticipate all that we shall learn today, but I think a major fact that will emerge is that the methodology for determining benefit–risk ratios is yet to be fully defined. Perhaps in the next 10 or 20 years, or even sooner as a result of today's meeting, we may actually reach a stage when we can accurately assess benefits, however they are measured, whether clinical, economic or psycho–social, whether we are talking about extending life or looking at the quality of life. We need to find better ways and means of determining risks, whatever they might be, some overall measure of morbidity and mortality. As a result it may then be possible to plot on a matrix system (Figure 1) any new chemical entity

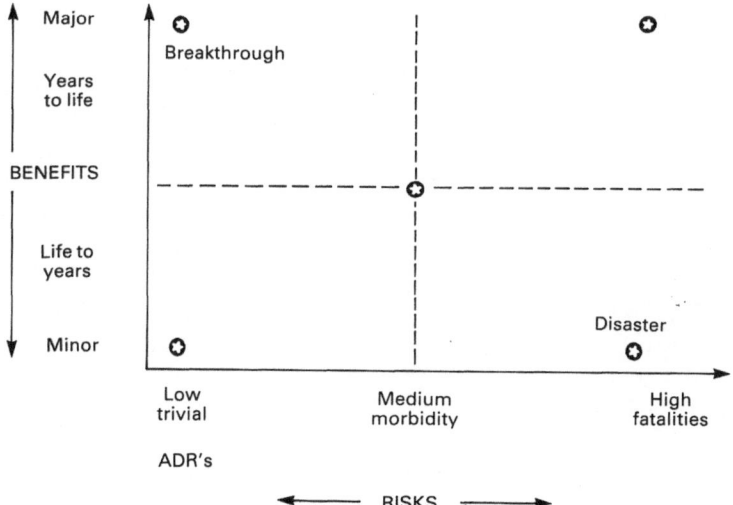

Figure 1 Medicines – the benefit–risk ratio (From *Pharm. J.*, 1986, **236**, 584, reproduced with permission)

1

at the product licence stage, or perhaps more importantly at a post-marketing stage. This figure tries to illustrate that a drug with major benefits and low side-effects might be classed as a breakthrough, whereas a medicine with very minor benefits but high fatalities or high risks, is classified as a disaster. All drugs lie somewhere within this matrix.

I am sure we shall find out today whether or not this is feasible, achievable or if there is any way in which we could work towards this end. I am delighted that so many eminent people have agreed to spend a day discussing the important subject of medicines and risk–benefit decisions.

Session 1

Risks in Perspective

1.1 The risks in society

Professor T. R. Lee

My emphasis will be on the perception of risks within society, particularly the very rapidly changing attitudes that are developing towards risk itself. At the moment my principal research activity is concerned with public attitudes towards ionizing radiation, and four major sites in Britain, where radioactive waste is to be disposed of or stored, are to be announced shortly. There will be a considerable public reaction to the threatened risk, in spite of an immense amount of scientific evidence that ionizing radiation can be adequately controlled and does not present risks comparable to many other energy sources. For example, the Outward Bound scheme killed 12 people in 8 years, but so far as we know there have been no deaths directly attributable to ionizing radiation in this country. So there is a paradox presented by extreme public attitudes of opposition and of complacency towards the risks presented within society. There is also a growing mistrust of scientific expertise, which needs to be considered very carefully.

The burgeoning concern over risks and hazards arising from technology is not easily explained. The conditions in Western civilization today are probably the safest that have ever existed, but in spite of this people get extremely worried. This is partly a result of technology, which has effectively controlled many minor risks, leaving disasters uncontrolled. It is the disasters or catastrophes that the public worries about, particularly because these are man-made and no longer 'natural'. One of the difficulties is that society, at least partially, is being converted to the concept of scientific determinism. Religion, magic, or fatalism are no longer relied upon to explain the disasters that occur because it is assumed that all disasters or events have causes, a view not wholly contributed to by scientists. This leads psychologists to study 'attribution theory', which is the attribution of responsibility for accidents.

There is also a moral concern about the future of society, with those who would like to revert to a 'state of nature' and those who see, on the contrary, that perhaps technology has the capacity to solve the problems that it creates. This is the attitude towards technology which might be characterized as the 'technological fix'.

Public attitudes towards risk present some bizarre anomalies. One that is relevant to today's discussions is that 2500 times as much money is spent on safety in the pharmaceutical industry as is spent on safety in the agricultural industry. It costs £1000 to dispose of one 200 litre can containing very low level radioactive waste, because of public anxieties which run far ahead of objective and scientific evidence. It cost the country £20m initially to save a life in the Ronan Point tower-block disaster, although shortly before that the WHO had pointed out that US$15 would save a life from smallpox, and currently a very small amount would save a child from death by dehydration in underdeveloped countries.

These are instances in which the public has a discrepant view from science that is vastly exaggerated, but there are also areas of incredible complacency. For example, approximately 1000 lives could readily have been saved last year with the imposition of a cervical screening service, at a very small cost. The public has a trusting faith in the engineering industry although one hundred dams collapsed during the period 1930–1980 and 15–16% of bridges collapse in the course of construction. There is, therefore, much anomaly which requires explanation.

The pharmaceutical industry engages in 'technological fixes', endlessly trying to improve the science without beginning to understand that what is primarily involved is public attitudes. There is a public outcry over relatively minor side-effects and the relatively small number of deaths, but the public does not pay corresponding attention to the infinite number of benefits that may be accrued from medicines. The industry in turn does not communicate to the public the possibility of weighing the risks against the benefits in any kind of rational way, and this only serves to accelerate an ever downward path in which more and more is spent on the 'techno-logical fix' which yields fewer and fewer benefits.

The scientific methods used to make predictions about the risks associated with different medicines are severely limited, in the sense that they concentrate on very speculative science, making generalizations usually from animals. When extrapolations are being made from human mortality it is deaths that are considered because they are readily measured. Many of the other side-effects, which are often of concern to the public, are less tangible and difficult to quantify.

Scientists are self-selected by predisposition to particular points of view and they become more converted to these points of view by their affilia-tions, the source of their income and their professional and formative pressures. Therefore, I am not surprised to discover that the speaker at a conference who states that 'the toxic risks from heavy metals are greatly exaggerated' comes from Rio Tinto Zinc or that the speaker who states that 'the risks from nuclear power stations are greatly exaggerated' comes from the Central Electricity Generating Board. The fact that people self-select themselves into different kinds of situations and then progressively make constructions of reality that accord with their self-interest is a psychological observation with a great deal of supporting evidence.

There is now an emerging science concerned with the objective observation of public attitudes towards hazards and risks. By comparing the perceived severity of different risks it becomes possible to 'unpack' the complex set of attributes that people attached to particular hazards. There is a chapter in the recent Royal Society Study Group publication on the perception of risk which refers to this[1].

The first step in this kind of comparison is to take a set of risks and ask

Table 1 Ordering of perceived risk for 30 activities and technologies
(The ordering is based on the geometric mean risk ratings within each group. Rank 1 represents the most risky activity or technology)

	League of Women Voters	College students	Active Club members	Experts
Nuclear power	1	1	8	20
Motor vehicles	2	5	3	1
Handguns	3	2	1	4
Smoking	4	3	4	2
Motorcycles	5	6	2	6
Alcoholic beverages	6	7	5	3
General (private) aviation	7	15	11	12
Police work	8	8	7	17
Pesticides	9	4	15	8
Surgery	10	11	9	5
Fire fighting	11	10	6	18
Large construction	12	14	13	13
Hunting	13	18	10	23
Spray cans	14	13	23	26
Mountain climbing	15	22	12	29
Bicycles	16	24	14	15
Commercial aviation	17	16	18	16
Electric power (non-nuclear)	18	19	19	9
Swimming	19	30	17	10
Contraceptives	20	9	22	11
Skiing	21	25	16	30
X-rays	22	17	24	7
High school and college football	23	26	21	27
Railroads	24	23	20	19
Food preservatives	25	12	28	14
Food colouring	26	20	30	21
Power mowers	27	28	25	28
Prescription antibiotics	28	21	26	24
Home appliances	29	27	27	22
Vaccinations	30	29	29	25

Source: Slovic et al. (1980)[2]

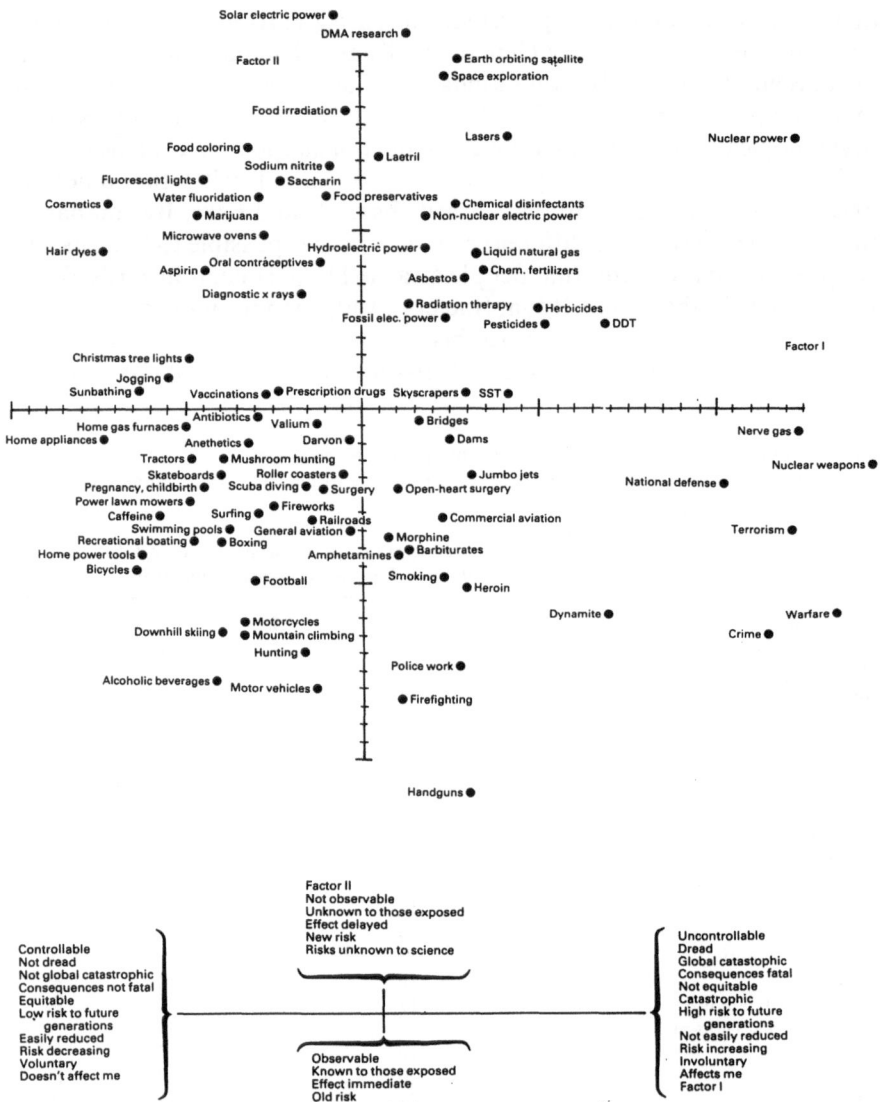

Figure 2 Hazard locations on Factors 1 and 2 of the three-dimensional structure derived from the interrelationships among 18 risk characteristics. Factor 3 (not shown) reflects the number of people exposed to the hazard and the degree of one's personal exposure. The diagram beneath the figure illustrates the characteristics that comprise the two factors. Source: Slovic *et al.* 1980[2]

people to assess them comparatively. A simple uni-dimensional measure of severity is used. This can then be pursued into a comparison between the severity as perceived by different groups as shown in Table 1. It will be found, for example, that nuclear experts place nuclear power twentieth in perceived severity, whereas the League of Women Voters put it first, as do students. Experts and students, both presumably with some scientific knowledge, rate food preservatives as more hazardous than do the League of Women Voters and others.

Next, by using a technique called 'factor analysis', the qualities of these perceived risks can be 'unpacked', as shown in Figure 2. People are asked to assess different hazards as, for example, controllable, uncontrollable, dreaded, global, catastrophic, equitable, inequitable, not easily reduced and so on. The principle of this analysis is to isolate the basic underlying dimensions, factors, or principal components. It is a statistical technique, and by asking people to evaluate each of the hazards on a wide range of attributes the main attribute dimensions are isolated. In Figure 2 they range from 'known' to 'unknown' and from 'not dreaded' to 'dreaded'. This is illustrated by the position of nuclear power, which indicates that the public perceives nuclear power at the extremes of these two principal dimensions. It is extremely severe with potential catastrophic implications and extremely unknown. Another dimension which has been isolated is that between small and large scale events.

The variables that mediate between the objective scientific computation of a risk and the public perception of that risk can be characterized in terms shown in Table 2.

Table 2   Variables that mediate between objective and perceived risk

Voluntary	Involuntary
Familiar	Unknown
Immediate	Delayed effect
Threat to self	Threat to society
Catastrophic	Chronic
Fates 'Worse than Death'	Clean, sharp death

Voluntary/involuntary – No-one would engage involuntarily in hang-gliding, but people are willing to take part in this type of activity because it is voluntary. In contrast, things such as nuclear power and chemical additives are beyond voluntary control and cause great concern.

Familiar/Unknown – Familiarity is a very important variable. Continuing exposure does not lead automatically to adaptation, but with prolonged exposure the perception of the risk and circumstances have changed to render them more tolerable.

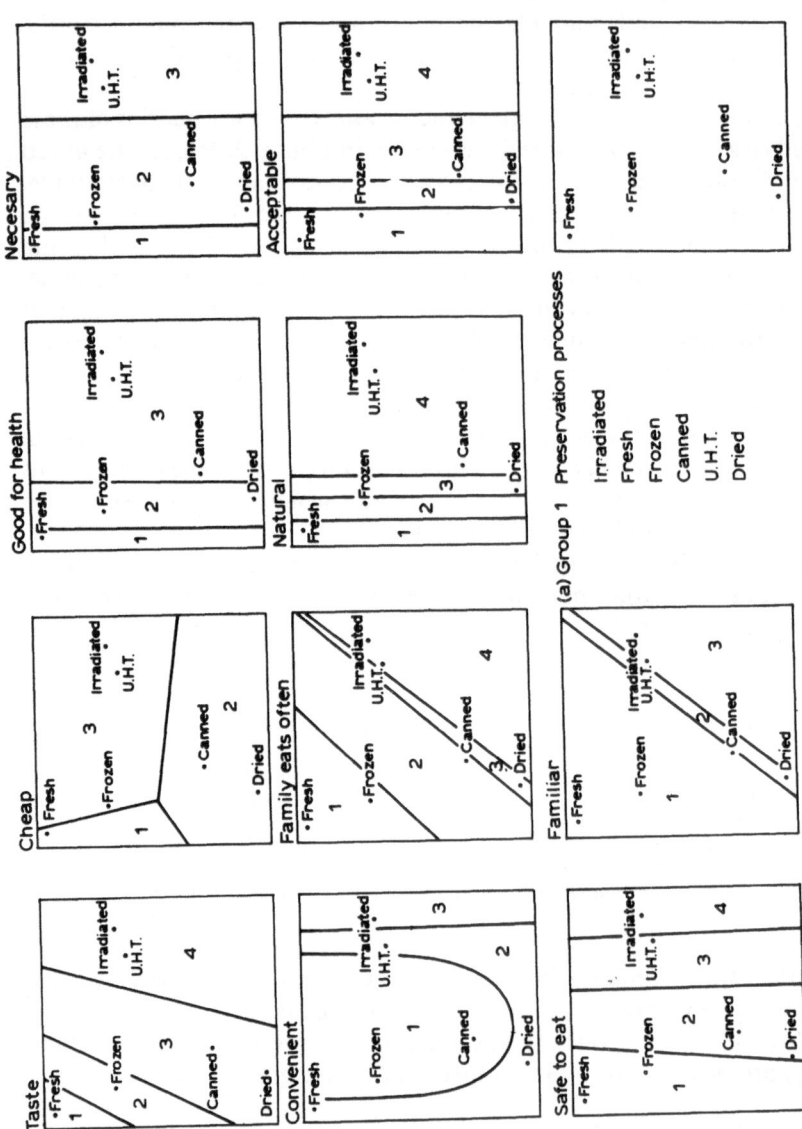

Figure 3   Multiple scalogram analysis of perceived safety with other attributes of food preservation processes.   Source: Lee (1986)[4]

Threat to self/threat to society – Nuclear power is perceived mainly as a moral threat to the future of civilization rather than as a threat to personal safety. For motorcycling or rock climbing the perception is of danger to self.

Catastrophic/chronic – If ten people die simultaneously in a disaster this is perceived as being more serious than if ten people die throughout the course of one year.

Multidimensional scaling analysis is another way of 'unpacking' the complexities of people's attitudes. I shall refer, finally, to a study conducted to explore how people perceive chemical food additives, food preservatives and substitute food substances[3,4]. This method takes care of the important point that 'riskiness' or 'safety' are attributes that do not exist in isolation – they are always synergistic with other perceived attributes of a hazardous technology or activity.

The approach illustrates a possible way ahead in exploring the public's changing attitudes towards medicines of different kinds.

The subjects, in this case a sample of 200 drawn from the general public, were asked to assess six additives, preservatives and substitutes, each on ten relevant attributes. They made their assessments on a 5 point scale. The resulting matrices are analysed (using the Guttman–Lingoes MDS Programme[5] in such a way that a single resolution into a two-dimensional space, incorporating the interactive influence for all ,the attributes, is arrived at. In statistical terms, the procedure is first to compute all the intercorrelations and then to produce an optimal arrangement of the items (i.e. food preservatives) as points in space, such that (a) proximity of the points represents *perceived similarity* on all the attributes and distance equals *dissimilarity*. (b) 'class membership' is preserved so that it is possible to display how each attribute has exercised its influence.

Only the results for food preservatives can be reproduced here as an example (see Figure 3). The strength with which each of the attributes is perceived to apply to a given preservative is given by the large numerals (1 = strong: 4 = weak). Hence, similarity if represented by the Euclidian distance between two points and the direction of influence by each attribute is represented by the vector formed from 1 to 4 as the space is partitioned. For example, it will be seen that canned and dried methods of preservation are perceived overall as relatively similar to each other and both are different from UHT and irradiated. The qualities of naturalness, safety and adaptability are perceived in much the same way – i.e. in a linear trend from fresh to irradiated; but cheapness has a non-linear relationship which arises from the perceived high cost of frozen food. Groups of medicines, for example tranquillizers, anti-depressants, β-blockers or analgesics, could be analysed in a similar way to determine what attributes the public applies to them and also what beliefs they have about them.

The terms risk and benefit come from economic modelling, which has dominated much of our research. They are usually restricted to things which are quantifiable, but these are not the most important things. It is important to determine people's beliefs about medicines and to find out how these beliefs combine to form their overall attitude.

References

1. Royal Society (1983). The perception of risks. Chapter V. In *Risk Assessment: A Study Group Report*. (London: Royal Society of London)
2. Slovic, P., Fischhoff, B. and Lichtenstein, S. (1980). Perceived risk. In R.C. Schwing and W.A. Albers (Eds) *Societal Risk Assessment: How Safe is Safe Enough?* (New York: Plenum Press)
3. Lee, T.R., Cody, C. and Plastow, E. (1985). Consumer attitudes towards technological innovations in food processing. (To be published)
4. Lee, T.R. Public attitudes towards chemical hazards. *Science of the Total Environment*, 51, 125–147
5. Lingoes, J.C. (1973). The Guttman Lingoes Nonmetric Program Series. Ann Arbor, University of Michigan, MA Thesis

1.2 The risks from diseases

Professor A. Smith

Disease is most conveniently defined as that which impairs or threatens to impair the individual's capacity to satisfy the requirements or to enjoy the rewards of an acceptable role within society. Such conditions may arise from innate anatomical or physiological disorders or from environmental insults of many different kinds, and may vary in severity from the trivial to the lethal and in duration from the transient to the permanent. The diversity of disease poses considerable problems for one who seeks to characterize its risks. To a considerable extent, the medical profession defines as diseases, those conditions which call for medical intervention designed to alleviate, contain or reverse their effects. This operational definition more or less defines the scope of available information, since the principal data source for statistics of disease is the records of the encounters of sick people with the medical services.

Illness is a widely dispersed feature of human existence even when operationally defined as above. Few people escape consultation with the medical services for more than a year at a time, and even fewer escape the need to negotiate some modification of their responsibilities because of less than optimal health. A substantial proportion of the population are restricted in their capacity to perform social roles as a result of more or less permanent health impairment. Nevertheless, we tend to define as serious diseases those conditions which are capable either of causing death or of restricting an individual's capacity for gainful employment for a substantial period of time. For most living creatures, life is beset with an almost continuous sequence of hazards in which injury, disability and eventually death are ultimately inevitable outcomes. The process of fertilization is itself a lottery, and each cell division which follows is associated with the possibility of errors which are potentially lethal, not only to the daughter cells but to the organisms of which they form a part. Some risks are innate consequences of the phenomenon of life and growth, some are more particular to individuals carrying known or

unknown mutant genes, some are characteristic of particular environmental experiences.

For humans, the risks have been brought under purposeful control to
an extent probably unique in the living world, a consequence – or possibly
a cause – of our unique conscious awareness of the dangerous nature of
existence. To some extent, we have achieved the possibility of choosing
between alternative hazards, and to some very small extent we are able to
make our choices on the basis of an understanding of relative risks. Nevertheless, most humans confront the hazards of their lives largely by
ignoring them, and we mostly live our lives as though they will never end.
This is partly because we differentiate a large number of risks with low
individual probabilities of occurrence, and partly because we are aware of
the enormous reductions in lethal risks that have been brought about
relatively recently.

The qualitative expression of risk becomes elusive when applied to an
individual, since individuals either incur a hazard or avoid it; the notion is
more tractable as well as more profitable when applied to a population.
Few would doubt that a proportion of the population will die in the
coming year, and experience persuades us that the proportion dying next
year will closely approximate the proportion that died last year.
Discernible trends usually continue, and in the absence of some special
knowledge of forthcoming changes in the population's general experience
predictions based on careful analysis of the past enjoy general credence.
Indeed, appropriately specific analysis of sub-categories of both the
population and the general disease experience enjoys a substantial
respectability as a predictive procedure with well established credentials.

Epidemiology is the science which is substantially concerned with
identifying and interpreting associations between the risk of disease or its
complications, and the personal, environmental and social experience of
those at risk. The quantitative expression of degree of risk usually
involves a ratio, and a very wide range of ratios has been used to suit
different purposes and to reflect different kinds of data. All ratios
represent a numerator divided by a denominator, and much of the
methodological pre-occupation of the epidemiologist is with selecting
appropriate numerators and denominators and obtaining reliable values
for them.

INCIDENCE AND PREVALENCE

Numerators for risk ratios may represent either a number of incidents (or
'events' to avoid the close homophony of 'incidents' and 'incidence') or a
number of individuals exhibiting some ascertainable attribute or state.
These two types of numerator require different types of denominator, and

the resulting ratios are distinguished as incidence and prevalence, respectively. Prevalence is the simpler concept. A prevalence ratio will have for its numerator the number of individuals found to exhibit some attribute or state, while the denominator will be a related number of individuals comprising both those so ascertained and those not so ascertained.

When individuals are examined for the presence of an ascertainable characteristic, the ratio of those found to have the characteristic to all those examined is the prevalence of the characteristic. Thus if 10% of examined individuals are found to have dental caries the prevalence of caries, at examination, is 10%. 'At examination' defines a point in time to which the prevalence refers. A prevalence 'point' may be in historical time (e.g. a date) or it may be a point in the lives of those under examination – such as 'at examination', 'at birth', 'at age 60' or 'at death'. Thus, the proportion found positive at cervical cytological examination, the stillbirth 'rate', the proportion of those with abnormal ECGs at their 60th birthday or the proportion of autopsy examinations in which the prostate is enlarged, are all prevalence ratios. Similarly, the proportion of the population resident in hospital on a census date is a prevalence ratio.

The numerator of an incidence rate will be a number of events incurred during a period of time, while the denominator will be the population at risk during the period. Often this will be estimated as the mid-point population. Incidents (events) may be disease onsets, consultations admissions, discharges, births, deaths or other events of medical or public health significance capable of being incurred by a population. The time base of an incidence must always be stated: for example, the crude death rate in the UK is about 12 per 1000 per year or 1 per 1000 per month. Just as the point in time to which the prevalence ratio is referred to may be in secular time or in life time, so the periods for incidence may be secular or part of the lifespan.

Prevalence is an appropriate measure of the burden of disease on a community at some point in time or stage of its experience. Incidence measures the intensity per unit time of the population's exposure to some category of event. For both, the reliable quantification of both numerators and denominators is the major pre-requisite.

Although prevalence ratios and incidence rates are quite different, and express different aspects of risk, there is clearly a relationship between them. For any state that is compatible with continued existence, its prevalence must be determined by the antecedent incidence of entry to the state and its characteristic duration. Generally speaking, prevalence is the product of the incidence of entry to the state and its duration, when the latter is measured in units of time base of the incidence rate. For example, if a disease has an annual onset incidence of two per 1000 persons and an average duration of 3 years, the prevalence at any point of time will be six per 1000 persons. Thus if the annual incidence of breast cancer is about 1 per 1000 women and the duration of the pre-symptomatic course averages 3 years, we should expect an efficient pre-symptomatic screening procedure to detect three cases per 1000 women examined. Clearly the duration of a state is itself a function of the incidence rates for entry to and exit from the state, but it is important to note that the denominators of the two incidences are different. For a state that is irreversible the incidence rate of exit is zero.

COMPARATIVE RISKS

If the annual incidence or the prevalence of a disease in a population exposed to a possible aetiological factor is 5% but only 1% in an unexposed population, the relative risk in the exposed population is 5-fold, and would usually be taken seriously as a potentially causal factor on the basis of such a relative risk. If the annual incidence (or the prevalence) were 24% in the exposed and 20% in the unexposed, the factor would probably be taken less seriously as a causal agent. Yet the *excess* morbidity attributable to the factor is 4% in each case and its significance to the population is equally great. Removal of the differential would be equally beneficial whether it changed the risk from 5% to 1% or from 24% to 20%. the 'attributable' risk associated with a factor may, therefore, be more important than the relative risk, although less persuasive of aetiological significance.

An interesting example of this distinction is the high relative risk of lung cancer associated with cigarette smoking and the low relative risk of ischaemic heart disease from the same cause. Nevertheless, the cardiovascular consequences of cigarette smoking are probably more important than the lung cancer risk because the attributable difference in mortality from heart disease is greater than that from lung cancer.

In contrast to both these ways of assessing different risks, it seems possible that the individual citizen prefers to compare the chances of avoiding an unfavourable outcome. For a disease whose risk is 5% and 1% in two different situations the chance of avoiding it is 95% and 94% – which may seem trivial as would a difference of 80% and 76%.

These different perspectives illustrate the need for caution in using the proportional experience of populations as guides to the significance of risk determinants. The aetiologist, the public policy maker and the individual may have different perceptions and different orders of priority.

A more striking example of the difference in viewpoint appropriate to the individual and to the community arises from what Rose[1] has called 'the prevention paradox'. The risk of cardiovascular or cerebrovascular death is related to arterial pressure level, just as the risk of perinatal death is related to birth weight, and the risk of alcohol-related disease is related to alcohol consumption. But the majority of cases of untoward outcomes occur to individuals occupying the centre rather than the extremes of the risk factor distributions, and the community's gain from a general shift of the centre of the distribution would be much greater than from any truncation of its tail. Thus the community's risk is not necessarily best improved by the simple aggregate of the responses appropriate to the individual's risks. Mortality associated with arterial pressure levels would be significantly improved by measures capable of lowering mean population pressures by 5 mmHg rather than by a treatment capable of lowering pressure in hypertensive by 50 mmHg or more.

EFFECTS OF AGE

The incidence of most diseases differs with age. The reasons comprise a wide variety of biological, social and environmental determinants of disease development. Diseases which involve permanent states tend to show a rising prevalence with age, unless an accelerated mortality eliminates both numerator and denominator or unless incidence fails to continue through the lifespan. For example, the prevalence of accidentally induced limblessness increases with advancing age, whilst that of most congenital conditions declines with age.

One of the most striking phenomena of recent human history (i.e. the past 1000 years and especially the past 200 years) has been the profound reduction in mortality seen in the age range 5 to 50 years, and which is usually considered to be due to quite fundamental changes in the social, economic and physical environment. Most of the change took place before the middle of the nineteenth century although the improvements continued into the early part of the present century, since when most of the improvements have been seen in the age range 0 to 5 years.

The decline in mortality in early to middle life is more probably a recent phenomenon – that is, it is probably a characteristic of the last 1000 years, and probably took place mainly in the period between 1700 and 1900, since that is the period in which the populations of industrializing countries exhibited their most remarkable growth and at a time when birth rate was either stationary or declining. Relatively little fall in mortality has occurred during the present century in industrialized countries, and most of the modest fall that has taken place occurred during the first third of the century. It is interesting to note that most of the observed decline in mortality from infectious disease had already occurred before the introduction of chemotherapy or antibiotics. It should also be noted that the introduction of the NHS in 1948 was associated with a cessation of the fall in early mortality which had been proceeding relatively steadily since the early years of the century. This fall was resumed some 20 years later. Neither the technical ingenuity of medical practice nor its accessibility to the population seem to exert a markedly favourable influence on mortality trends.

The remarkable reduction in the risk of dying before the onset of what is considered to be old age has been accompanied by an equally remarkable absence of improvement in the risk of dying once old age is reached. Since environmental change is well established as the reason for the reduced risk at earlier ages it is natural to assume that the determinants of the risks of death in old age lie much less in the environment and possibly more in the human genotype. Indeed, some have suggested that the diseases which cause death in old age occur when they do precisely because our evolution has selectively eliminated genotypes associated with their earlier onset. This is tantamount to viewing these diseases as mechanisms by which our species characteristic lifespan is implemented, and tends to lead to the view that these diseases are unlikely to be preventable, and not readily curable.

Nevertheless, the diseases which predominate among the causes of death in old age – cancer, stroke, ischaemic heart disease – exhibit substantial evidence of environmental 'causation'. Most show striking secular and geographical variation in their distribution and for most, there is a considerable aetiological literature implicating the relevance of a range of environmental or behavioural variables. The challenge is to explain the concentration of disease occurrence in the older age groups, the relative intractability of these diseases to environmental improvement and often to therapeutic measures, and in many cases the wide range of aetiological variables with which they are associated.

The association of risk of many lethal diseases with advancing age has received considerable attention. The epithelial cancers – for which this association is particularly striking – have attracted the speculation of mathematicians who have fitted suitable curves to the available data and drawn aetiological inferences from their equations. The notion is now quite widespread that the appearance of these cancers is the outcome of a series of independent events each having a specifiable probability of occurrence (risk), but required to occur in the appropriate sequence in order to 'permit' the cancer to develop. The shape of the curves relating incidence or mortality to age are usually of the form:

$$\text{Incidence} = f(\text{age}^n) \text{ where } n \text{ is 5 or 6.}$$

From this it is often concluded that the causal sequence must contain five or 6 necessary factors occurring in the appropriate order.

However, much simpler and more plausible models are capable of explaining the observed associations. For example: if each citizen regularly received a premium bond and these were accumulated over the course of time, the distribution of prizes would exhibit an association with age of the general form observed with deaths from cancer, heart disease or stroke. Precise fits can be achieved by varying the rate of acquisition of bonds in simple linear ways. In other words, if a random event occurs to 'eligible' individuals and if the prevalence of the eligibility builds up as the cumulative incidence of access to the eligible state, the association of the event with age will exhibit the familiar relationship observed for many of the diseases characteristic of old age. If the incidence of onset of the eligible condition is variably associated with certain aetiological factors and if the probability of the 'random' event also varies with other associated factors, the simple 'premium bond' model can account for most of the observed associations with both age and aetiological factors.

The advantages of this model include its relative simplicity and its plausibility in terms of what we know of the epidemiology of the common fatal conditions. Perhaps more importantly, the model provides the possibility of a wide range of potential preventive or interventive strategies. Nevertheless, the possibility that many of the currently intractable disease problems may yield to intervention, raises new difficulties. Much of the relative intractability of these current problems is the consequence of our earlier success in eliminating those diseases which proved relatively easy to deal with. As each manageable problem is eliminated, so what remains becomes increasingly an intractable core. Much of the difficulty of present therapeutic problems is the consequence of earlier preventive success. This process is likely to continue so that each advance renders the residual problems more difficult. The challenge, both to the clinician and to the pharmaceutical industry, is likely to become increasingly formidable, and the responsibilities placed on a caring society will inevitably become increasingly onerous.

VARIATIONS IN DISEASE RISK IN EUROPE

World variations in disease experience are huge, and reflect both the variations in morbidity attributable to differences in climate, geography and social and political development and also to differences in mechanisms of data-capture. Within Europe some of the variation is more surprising in view of the relative social and geographical homogeneity of much of the region.

Expectation of life at birth (essentially the mean age at death) varies from 51.4 years to 73.5 for males and from 54.5 to 79.8 for females. This has generally increased by about 20 years during the present century but by much less during the past 25 years.

Infant mortality exerts the major effect on life expectancy and it is now as low as 8 per 1000 live births in the more favoured European countries.

It varies considerably both between and within European countries, showing marked differentials in this country across the social classes and between North and South. These gradients have changed very little since data have been available.

The lethal diseases of adult life exhibit remarkable variation among the countries of Europe (Table 3), and continue to suggest that there remains substantial room for progress even in our own country. At one time, mortality in England and Wales was among the lowest in the world – a situation which is decreasingly the case – especially for heart disease and cancer.

Table 3 Deaths per 100000 per annum, Males

	Age group	*Cancer*	*Heart disease*	*Violence*	*All causes*
England and Wales	15–24	8.3	—	60.5	87.7
Highest European		21.9	—	147.0	189.9
		(Luxemburg)		(Austria)	(Portugal)
Lowest European		7.5		35.6	87.4
		(Belgium)		(Malta)	(Malta)
England and Wales	25–44	28.9	43.4	42.8	141.6
Highest European		40.4	79.8	149.3	333.1
		(Czecho-slovakia)	(Hungary)	(Poland)	(Portugal)
Lowest European		12.2	26.7	41.8	123.8
		(Malta)	(Norway)	(Netherlands)	(Netherlands)
England and Wales	45–64	367.7	646.8	50.4	1,255.1
Highest European		425.5	857.4	206.5	1,592.6
		(Czecho-slovakia)	(Finland)	(Hungary)	(Finland)
Lowest European		248.1	307.8	40.7	826.5
		(Sweden)	(Greece)	(Malta)	(Greece)
England and Wales	65 & over	1,591.4	3,747.0	102.3	7,234.0
Highest European		1,868.8	5,833.3	426.0	8,666.7
		(Netherlands)	(Malta)	(Hungary)	(Malta)
Lowest European		820.0	2,399.8	133.3	4,880.0
		(Iceland)	(Greece)	(Malta)	(Iceland)

Source: Health Services in Europe, Vol 2 World Health Organisation, Regional Office for Europe, 1981.

The risks from diseases remain substantial, very variable and potentially amenable to improvement by rationally based interventions employing therapeutic agents, immunizing procedures, behavioural change and social and political actions. They constitute the major threat to the enjoyment of a long and full human life, and probably merit the acceptance of the generally smaller and more controllable risks associated with health and medical care.

Reference

1. Rose, G. (1981). Strategy of prevention: lessons from cardiovascular disease. *Br. Med. J.*, **282**, 1847-51

1.3 Perception of risk

Dr J. Urquhart

The public's perceptions of risk might be epitomized by the trick question that was popular when I was about 8 or 9 years old: which is heavier, a pound of feathers or a pound of lead? It is a question that loses its trick character after one has digested the basic idea of weights and measures, but is a distinct challenge to a mind that is in transition from ignorance to the understanding of these fundamentals.

In the public's perception of risks there are many examples which show confusion of the feathers/lead variety. These have been widely commented upon before[1-4] and Professor Lee's paper at this meeting summarizes them.

Before throwing up our hands at the hopeless and unpredictable inconsistencies of the public's responses to risk and risk-related information, we should take note of a fundamental element missing from this whole story. The fact is that no measure or scale for risk has public currency. Consequently, the vast majority of people are ill-informed about the magnitudes of risks that prevail in today's life. There is, to be sure, a vast amount of data available in actuarial and public health or other official reports, but these data are obscure, insofar as the general public is concerned. Moreover, the formatting of risk-related information in actuarial and official reports is not conducive to public communication: most of this data is reported in the format of '4.9 deaths per 100 000 per year'. Heilmann and I have dubbed this the 'epsykay pe-put' scale (*events* per one hundred thousand (*CK*, in roman numerals) *people per unit time*) and the deliberate absurdity of this name epitomizes the absurdity of trying to use the epsykay pe-put format in communicating risk-related information to the public.

It is not certain that public perceptions would improve if there existed a simple, widely-used scale for communicating risk-related information, but it is hard to see that matters could be worse with such a scale than without. If the analogy to the system of weights and measures has some validity, one may note that having a universal system of weights and measures has certainly not solved all the problems of trade, but it has served to purge the market-place of a basic confusion and mistrust about quantification of goods bought and sold.

RISK COMPARISONS

A widely-accepted scale is basic to comparing the risks posed by various of life's hazards. As Lord Rothschild pointed out in an especially lucid Dimbleby Lecture in 1978, risk comparisons are 'the best antidote to panic'[5] because they create a context for assessing the risk posed by a new or newly-discovered hazard with the risk posed by a familiar hazard.

I must reiterate the caution that having a widely accepted scale and a simple basis for risk comparisons will not create a populace of consistently strict rationalists. Yet the situation today is that most people over-estimate the small risks in life, and under-estimate the big ones[6,7]. In part, this prevailing misunderstanding is the consequence of a structural bias in news reporting, epitomized in the old journalists' law: 'man bites dog – that's news; dog bites man – that's not news'. Unfortunately, in reporting the rare man-bites and not reporting the frequent dog-bites, the public is misled to infer that man-bites outnumber dog-bites.

Pursuing the idea of risk comparisons from several different perspectives will serve to illustrate several alternative ways to communicate risk-related information.

Historical risk comparisons

In considering historical comparisons, one naturally should take into account the evolution of medical knowledge. A good starting point is a familiar piece of anecdotal Victorian art, Sir Luke Fildes's *The Doctor* (1891), which hangs in the Tate Gallery. It shows a wise-looking, frock-coated, graying medical man sitting pensively, and perhaps prayerfully, at the side of a makeshift bed in which lies a sick little girl; the anxious parents hold each other in the background shadows of the room, and some inconsequential liquid medicine sits on a table, almost out of the picture. This painting epitomizes the practice of medicine at the turn of the century, just before the chemical industry began to invest in research on pharmaceuticals. David Rutstein, who taught me preventive medicine at Harvard, used to say that this was when a house-call cost 50 cents, and that was about all it was worth!

The contemporary version of Fildes's painting would show a very different scene, with an active doctor using powerful drugs, techniques,

and devices, coupled with a level of sanitation and hygiene that was still
not widely practised in 1891. Also, the patient hovering at death's door
would more typically be an old lady rather than a little girl.

When I last visited the Tate, *The Doctor* happened to be featured as the
'picture of the month' and thus the subject of a daily lecture; this attracted
a large audience whose main interest seemed much less the artistic aspects
of the work than nostalgia for the warm and caring style of medical
practice it depicted. It was quite clear that few admirers of the scene
comprehended that the turn-of-the-century doctor was an ineffectual
witness who brought little more to the scene than a taxonomy for
classifying diseases and some micro-organisms from his previous patients.

A more quantitative view of historical risk comparisons comes in
looking at survival curves across the decades. Figure 4 shows one of the
earliest sets of such data, from Breslau (now Wroclaw) in 1690, compared
with two curves for Americans born in 1907. The lower curve for 1907,

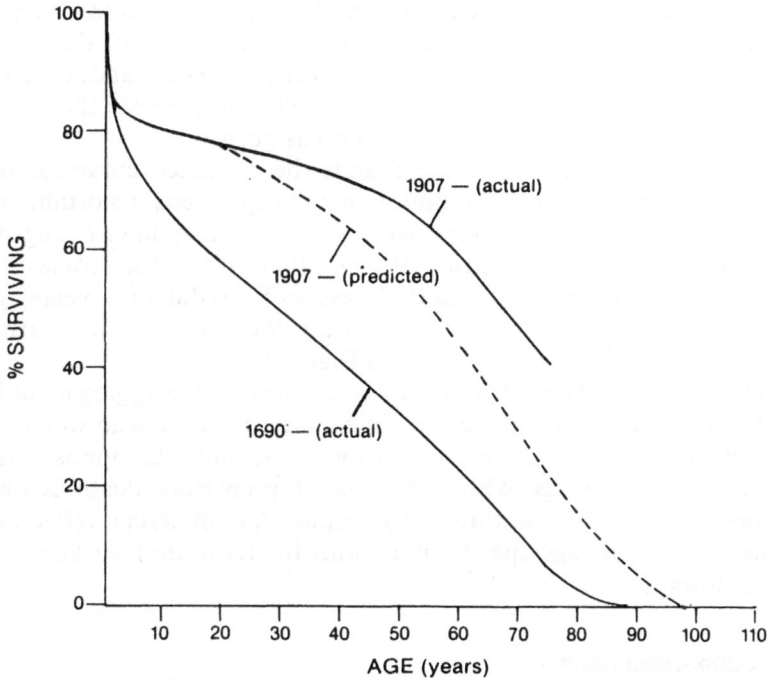

Figure 4 The percentage of survivors of those born in any year declines steadily with
age. The line labelled '1907 – (actual)' was drawn in 1984 based on data for survivorship of Americans born in 1907. The line labelled '1907 – (predicted)' was derived by
applying the age-specific mortality rates prevailing in 1906 to Americans born in 1907.
The line labelled '1690 – (actual)' is based on contemporary data from the city of
Breslau (Wroclaw). This figure is reproduced, with permission, from Reference 8, which
documents the sources of these curves

labelled 'predicted', is a forecast based on the assumption that people born in 1907 would be subject, throughout their lives, to the age-specific mortality rates that had prevailed in 1906; in other words, a prediction based on there being neither advances nor setbacks in public health after 1906. The upper curve shows the actual survivorship of the 1907 cohort. People born in 1907 lived longer than they were projected to at the time of their birth, and a much larger fraction of those born in 1907 lived into their early and later adult years than people had back in the 17th century. It is also noteworthy that the people born in 1907 have survived much better than they were predicted to, notwithstanding the fact that their lives coincided with the vast proliferation of automobiles, synthetic chemicals, complex industries and their effluvia, powerful drugs with sometimes lethal side-effects, and all the other sometimes frightening aspects of life that the code-words 'pollution' and 'unrestrained technology' may conjure.

The shape of the survival curve for the 1907 cohort is not unique, for the curves of other years in the early part of this century would also have a similar shape. By this I specifically mean that the slopes of the survival curves at each age of life for those born in other years are about the same as the slopes for the 1907 cohort. I chose 1907 to illustrate these points only because that was the year my father was born.

Going one step further, Figure 5 adds the predicted curve for those born in 1977, based on the assumption that the age-specific mortality rates of 1976 would not change. We already know that they have changed for the better in Western countries, though slightly for the worse in the Eastern bloc[9]. One might hazard the guess, as Fries did a few years ago[10], that the actual curve for those born in the West in 1977 may turn out something like the uppermost curve in Figure 5.

From this historical view, one may conclude that the aggregate of life's lethal risks are at an historical low. In contrast to those who would have us believe that we live in uniquely risky times, quite the opposite is the case: we live in an age where the risk of premature death is unprecedentedly low, and is continuing to decline. A commercial reflection of this fact is that the age-specific premiums for term life insurance are at historic lows[11].

Unprecedented risks

One may reasonably enquire how the always possible threat of unprecedented disaster influences the reckoning of risk in today's life. Such threats include the traditional four apocalyptic events: war (nuclear or other), pestilence (AIDS or other), famine and natural disasters (fire, flood, earthquake, etc.). The answer is that the history of such disasters on a large scale shows them to be so infrequent as to be projected as having a tiny

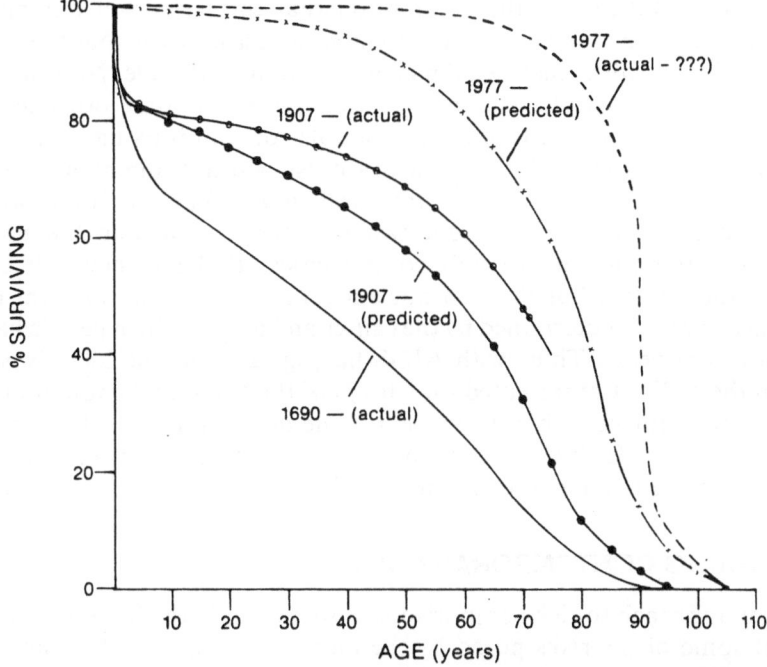

Figure 5 The 1690 (actual), 1907 (actual) and 1907 (predicted) curves are the same as in Figure 4. The curve labelled '1977 – (predicted)' is based on the assumption that Americans born in 1977 will face the age-specific mortality rates that prevailed in the US during 1976. The curve labelled '1977 – (actual) – ???' is only a guess at what the future might bring, assuming that (1) war, pestilence, or famine do not overtake us; (2) progress continues. This figure is reproduced, with permission, from Reference 8, which documents the sources of these curves

probability of occurring presently or in the near future. As the recent disastrous earthquakes in Mexico show, however, 'tiny probability' does not mean zero probability, zero risk, or absolute safety. By comparison, there are two million deaths annually in the USA, the vast majority of which result from one of the following: coronary heart disease, cancer, stroke, respiratory diseases, motor vehicle accidents, falls, liver disease, complications of diabetes and suicide. Thus, the probability of one's dying in a big disaster is vastly overshadowed by the probability of death from one of the above-listed causes.

A logical, but not necessarily emotionally compelling, corollary of the foregoing is that the antecedent 'risk factors' for these common causes of death are natural foci of risk-related concerns, both for individuals and society.

What one calls 'risk' for the purpose of pricing term life insurance is based on extrapolating the experience of the near-term past to projecting the near-term future, on the assumption that the latter will not differ drastically from the former. It is in this same actuarial sense that I use the work 'risk' here, with 'near-term' meaning roughly a decade. No-one can guarantee that war will not occur, or that AIDS or some other lethal disease will not continue to annually double (or more) its incidence, or that some great upheaval of the earth's crust will not annihilate whole regions, or that vast crop failures will not occur, or that some unprecendented geothermal event will not happen, melting the polar icecap and flooding the world's coastal cities. Perhaps they will and perhaps they won't, but they do not enter into the pricing of term life insurance, which is determined by the causes and ages at which people have died in recent years. Thus, with AIDS having taken about 2000 lives in 1984 in the US[12], it represented only 0.1% of the total, and could double annually for four years before exceeding the death toll in the US due to drunk driving[13,14] for example, or for eight years before approaching the death toll in the US due to cigarette smoking[15].

COMPARING CONTEMPORARY RISKS

Another approach to risk comparisons, anticipated in the foregoing, is to look at some of the risks posed by the more widely-accepted hazards in everyday life.

Figure 6 shows American mortality due to car accidents in relation to overall mortality at different ages. For people in their early twenties, it accounts for almost half the deaths. Of course, not very many people die in their twenties, so Figure 6 does have have a certain alarmist quality when viewed out of context with, for example, Figure 5.

There is a pharmacological element in these car-crash fatalities, as Figure 7 shows. During the night-hours, when the vast majority of fatal accidents occur, the blood alcohol level is over the legal limit in about $\frac{3}{4}$ of the fatally-injured car drivers, and most experts maintain that strict separation of driving and drinking would halve the traffic death toll [13, 14]. Figure 8 shows, however, that the fatally-injured drivers are not alone in their immediately ante-mortem consumption of alcohol: about $\frac{5}{8}$ of pedestrians fatally injured during the night-hours were themselves drunk at the time. These data do not, *per se,* establish causality and beg to be supplemented, for example by measures of the prevalence of high blood-alchohol levels among those who were able to make their way home safely.

A rather compelling answer to the question of the causal role of excessive alcohol intake in premature death comes from the life insurance industry. A practical, if unscientific, guide to the overall mischief of alcohol (Table 4) has been provided by Brackenridge[19]. Brackenridge was medical director of a leading British life insurance firm, and has summarized his experience in how to adjust life insurance premiums in

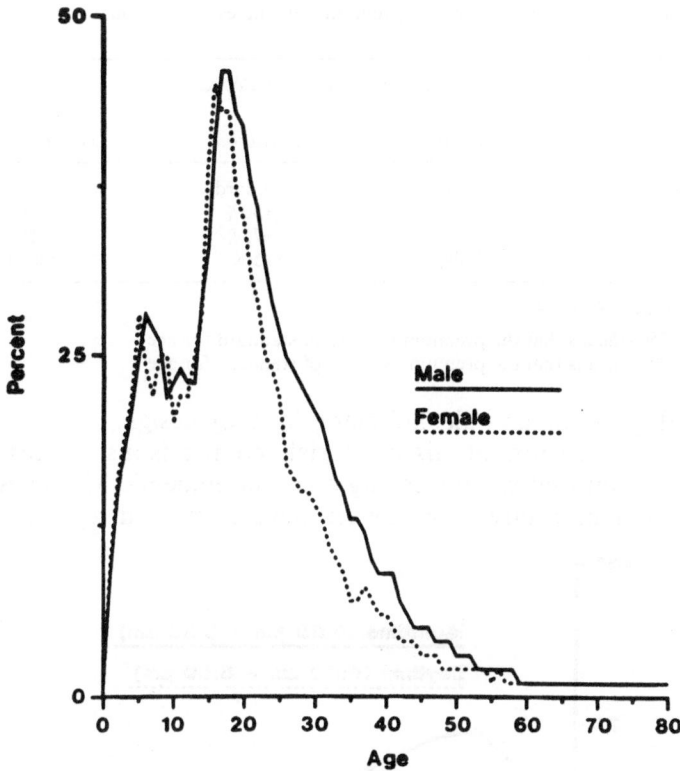

Figure 6   The proportion of deaths in the US at each age due to automobile accidents for the year 1978. Reproduced, with permission, from Reference 16, which documents the sources of the data

the light of a whole panoply of medical considerations, including the applicant's drinking history. While not the results of a carefully controlled clinical trial, Brackenridge's experience is one tempered by many years' experience with the economic discipline of pricing life insurance premiums and paying death claims. His overview, summarized in Table 4, is a semi-quantitative reinforcement of the exquisite literary cameo on alcohol that Alex Comfort recently published in *The Lancet*[20], and to Dame Sheila Sherlock's indictment[21] of the wrong-headedness in research funding that gives little support to better understanding of our most widely-used drug and its role as a major hazard in human life.

People schooled in contemporary precepts of clinical pharmacology will find various ways to fault the validity of Brackenridge's conclusions, but the discipline of steering between the alternative pitfalls of over- and under-pricing life insurance is an arguably good antidote to bias in a field

Table 4 Adjustments in life insurance premiums in males for various degrees of alcohol consumption

	Extent of alcohol's effect		
Frequency of occurrence	*Jovial*	*Boisterous*	*Uncontrolled*
6 Times/year	standard	standard	+50%
Monthly	standard	+50%	+100%
Weekly	+25%	+75%	+150%
Daily	+100%	+150%	decline

Source: Reference 19, p.734

Note: +25% means that the premium is 125% of standard for age
         +100% means that the premium is 200% of standard for age

ridden with pro- and anti-alcohol biases in study design.

Another dimension of historial risk comparisons relates to the prevalent notion that we are having a cancer epidemic. Of course, both incidence and mortality from cancer have a marked age-dependency

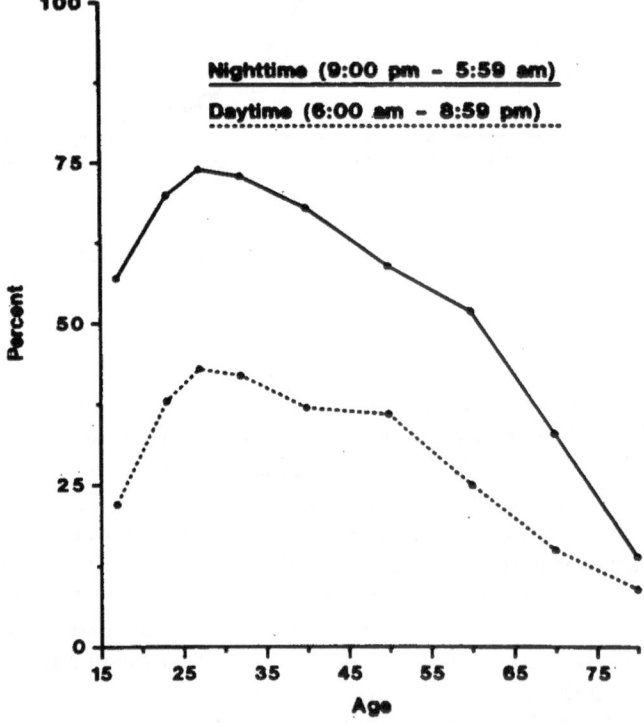

Figure 7 The proportion of fatally injured US motor vehicle drivers during 1979–81 whose blood alcohol levels exceeded the legal limit of 0.1 mg/100 ml. Reproduced, with permission, from Reference 17 which documents the sources of the data

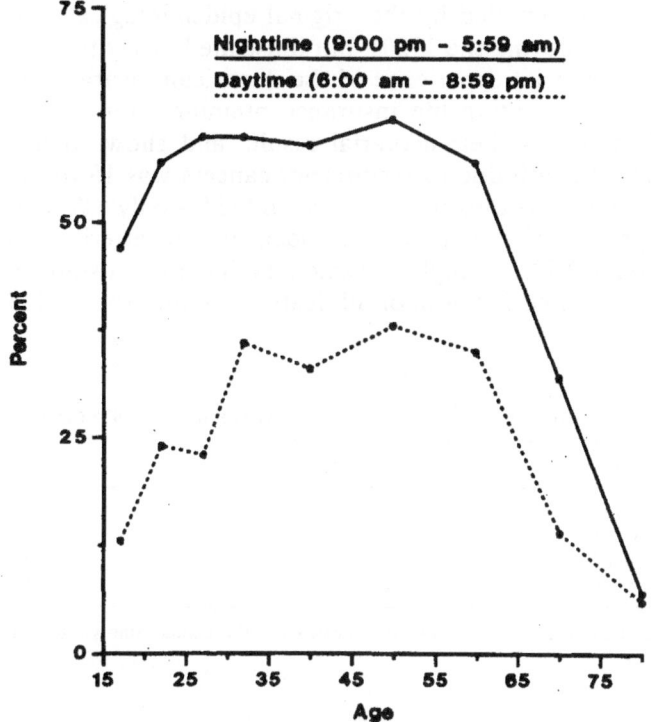

Figure 8 The proportion of fatally injured US pedestrians during 1979–81 whose blood alcohol levels exceeded 0.1 mg/100 ml. Reproduced, with permission, from Reference 18 which documents the sources of the data

(Table 5). Obviously, with an ageing population, the absolute numbers of cancer victims are rising. However, the historical trends in cancer mortality are quite otherwise when the ageing of the population is corrected for (Figure 9). Age-adjusted mortality is declining steeply for both uterine and stomach cancers, the former because of earlier diagnosis and better treatment, the latter for reasons unknown, but clearly not because of better treatment. The only 'cancer epidemic' we are seeing is of lung cancer and the basis for that in widely prevalent cigarette smoking is well documented[22].

Relative vs absolute risk

However, the link between smoking and lung cancer illustrates another point of public misunderstanding. The biggest risk of smoking is not lung cancer, as widely believed, but premature death due to arteriosclerotic heart disease, as revealed by the original epidemiological studies in the UK and the US during the 1950s, but illustrated nicely for our purposes here by the actuarial experience of the American insurance firm which pioneered in discounting life insurance premiums for non-smokers [23]. Table 6 summarizes their actuarial results and shows that, while the relative risk of death due to respiratory cancers was 15 times higher in smokers than in non-smokers, these accounted for only 6% of all deaths in both groups. The risk of premature death due to arteriosclerotic heart disease is 'only' 2.7 times higher in smokers than in non-smokers, but this condition accounted for 30% of all deaths in both groups. This point is

Table 5   Death rates from cancer among Americans by age and sex, 1975 (deaths per 100000)

Age	Male	Female
25–44	34	33
45–54	184	177
55–64	512	358
65 and older	1221	725

Source: US Bureau of the Census, statistical abstract of the United States 1981, Table 117

illustrative of how the concepts of relative and of absolute risk may confuse people, e.g. the prevailing view that the chief mischief of cigarette smoking is that it causes lung cancer.

Statements of relative risk are the outcome of the currently popular 'case-control' studies. These have become popular with epidemiologists in recent years, and results of such studies often receive attention from the news media when the nature of the risk factor is something in everyday life and when the size of the relative risk looks impressive. Such news stories are patently misleading when the absolute risks involved are tiny, and they undoubtedly contribute to the widespread public impression that we live in times when the risk of premature death is unprecedentedly high.

GLEANING MEDICAL KNOWLEDGE FROM INSURANCE DATA

Cowell and Hirst's actuarial study[23] of life-insured smokers vs non-smokers has provided not the first but one of the strongest pieces of evidence on the adverse effects of cigarette smoking. It captures the results of a very large 'experiment of nature' (Table 6), 718 deaths occurring within the 5-year period in which deaths were tabulated, among insured

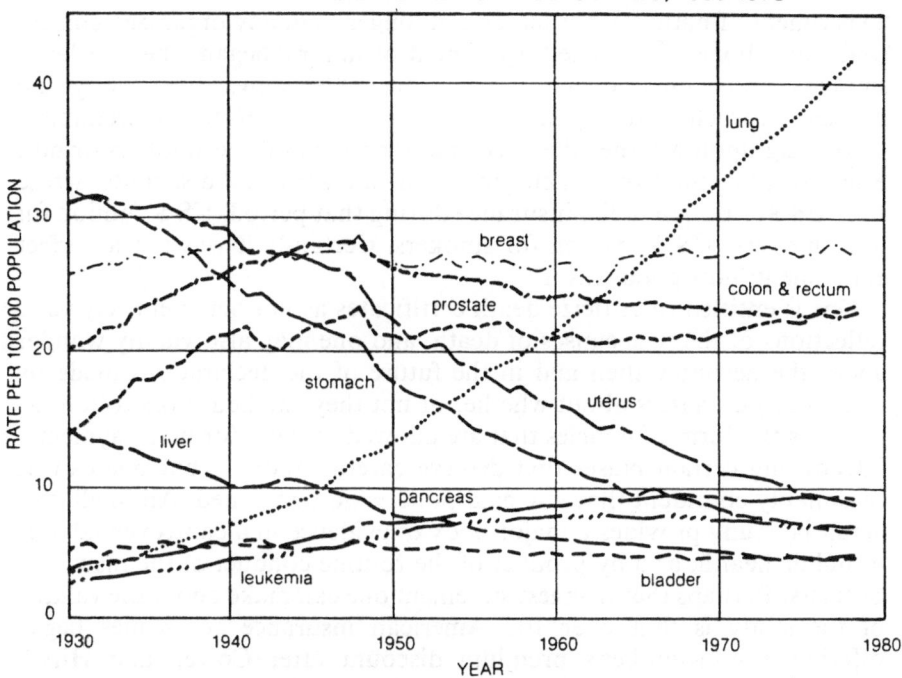

CANCER DEATH RATES BY SITE—UNITED STATES, 1930-1978

Rate for the population standardized for age on the 1970 U S population

Sources of Data National Center for Health Statistics and Bureau of the Census United States

Note Rates are for both sexes combined except breast and uterus female population only and prostate male population only

Figure 9   Changes in death rates from the various major types of cancer in the United States from 1930 to 1978. (Source: American Cancer Society, *Cancer Facts and Figures, 1983*. Reproduced with permission)

Table 6 State Mutual's experience based on 718 deaths among insured smokers and non-smokers, 1973-1978

% Deaths in categories	Cause of death	Ratio of death-risk smokers/non-smokers
100.0	All causes	2.2
6.0	Respiratory cancers	15.0
30.1	Arteriosclerotic heart disease	2.7
2.5	Hypertension and hypertensive heart disease	8.1
19.1	Cancer (excluding respiratory cancers)	1.2
4.9	Motor vehicle accidents	2.6
4.9	Suicide	9.0
32.5	All other	1.9

who had purchased their insurance as long ago as 15 years. As such, this 'experiment of nature' is far larger and longer than any organized clinical trial could hope to be. The 'experiment of nature' began when declared smokers and non-smokers opted, from 1965 onwards, to buy life insurance for which they paid somewhat different age-specific premiums, depending upon whether they declared themselves to be smokers or not. State Mutual, the firm which pioneered non-smokers' discounts, wrote over US $12 billion in life insurance during that period, US $7 billion for non-smokers, US $5 billion for smokers. Certainly it was not a perfect experiment; how good was it?

One is entitled to criticize death certificates as not being entirely valid reflections of the true causes of death, and one may also validly wonder about the accuracy then and in the future of the declarations made by insurance purchasers about whether or not they smoked. Loss to follow-up takes the form of policies that are allowed to lapse for non-payment – introducing certain biases that deserve careful study –– but one can be reasonably confident that few paid policies go unclaimed. All in all, this actuarial study provides a major body of evidence in a controversial area of public health, as a by-product of the routine conduct of the insurance business. Perhaps the strongest statement one can make about the validity of the study is that over 100 American insurance companies began offering a non-smoker's premium discount after Cowell and Hirst's actuarial study was published[24], signifying their confidence that this 'experiment' was repeatable.

It is well to recall that this is not the first time that important public health information has been a by-product of the actuarial analyses of the insurance industry. The big actuarial publication, *Build and Blood Pressure Study*[25], put an end to the myth of 'benign essential hypertension' that was standard medical teaching up until then. The 1959 study tabulated the actuarial consequences of having various degrees of elevated diastolic and/or systolic blood pressure. It was based on data from over 300000 people – another big 'experiment of nature', and it taught us doctors something about the natural history of a common human condition that we had previously misunderstood.

It seems fair to say that these big 'experiments of nature' are not ideal experiments, in the sense that we know in the contemporary methodology of clinical trials, but they have a very heavy weight of numbers and a long history of successfully guiding commercial decisions in the insurance industry – which speaks to their repeatability. Given the time, trouble, costs and sometimes disappointing outcomes of big clinical trials, I think we would do well to look carefully at the flow of information generated by the health and life insurance industry to see if it could not be more productively linked to the development of medical information on the long-term outcomes of therapeutic intervention.

DEFINING RISK

To clarify the semantics related to risk, it is useful to define (absolute) risk as: *the probability of occurrence of adversity within a defined time interval.* What the adversity is has to be specified, as does the time interval. This is not an idiosyncratic definition of risk but one that is now generally accepted[26]. Some would have it otherwise: a recent review in *Nature* of the book *Risk Watch*, stated: '... risk is only in a very limited sense a statistical concept. At its heart, risk is a culturally learned response to uncertainty ...'[27]. While such ideas may have a certain intuitive or emotional appeal, the simple fact is that the probabilistic definition of risk is numerically tractable, whereas the attempt to link probability and behavioural responses[28,29] is not.

One might analogously criticize the concept of the kilogram as being limited, for it does not extend to include the possible behavioural responses to, e.g. a kilogram of coal vs that of diamonds. Coal certainly has vast societal and political overtones as the British know only too well, as do diamonds, as the French and those interested in the socio-political scene in South Africa understand. Those are interesting possible extensions to the concept of 'kilogram', but to link them to the precisely defined concept of mass would destroy its numerical tractability and paralyse trade.

There is a good precedent in the insurance industry's risk assessment circle for the relatively recent meaning of 'risk' as being simply the probability of adversity and not some nebulous fusion of adversity's probability and severity. This precedent may be illustrated in the pricing of term life insurance, as follows. In general, one would consider the death of a 28-year-old father of four young children to be a considerably greater adversity than, for example, the death of a 78-year-old bachelor. The probabilities of death of the two differ by more than an order of magnitude, which fact is reflected in the standard tables of actuarial risk and thus in the pricing of term life insurance, which is straightforwardly linked to the age-specific annual probability of death. The prospective purchaser of life insurance can make his/her own reckoning about the severity of the adversity brought by death of the insured and can make a purchase decision against that reckoning, which is necessarily an individual matter. It would bring dreadful confusion to this rather straight-forward marketplace to introduce into the pricing of term life insurance an element reflecting the seller's pre-judgement about the purchaser's response to the uncertainty of death. So pricing relates strictly to probability, in a numerically tractable manner, and purchase decisions are made by individuals according to their own judgements about the nature and magnitude of the adversity for which they seek insurance.

COMMUNICATING ABSOLUTE RISK TO THE PUBLIC

There are a number of numerically equivalent ways to express risk, as defined. Among experts, the most common way is to use the epsykay-peput scale. That may be suitable for experts but it is not particularly helpful in communicating risk-related information to the general public, which is the main focus of this paper. Lord Rothschild pointed out that an equivalent but much simpler and more easily grasped format was to say 1 event in U people per unit time. In that format, the risk statement contains two pertinent numbers: (a) 1, which is an individual – you, me, whomever, but a single unlucky person; (b) U, which is the size of the group needed, on average, to produce one victim and which number Heilmann and I have termed the 'unicohort'[6,30].

Obviously, the bigger the unicohort, the smaller the risk and vice versa. The smallest conceivable unicohort is 1, which would be the case in describing a situation where adversity was inevitable, e.g. a suicidal leap from the Golden Gate Bridge. The largest potentially definable unicohort is half the population of the largest country that regularly collects and reports reliable data on its citizens' vital statistics – health, accidents, mortality, births and so forth. That country happens currently to be the United States, so that the largest potentially definable unicohort today is around 100 million. If the Chinese ever begin to collect and report reliable vital statistics, then the largest definable unicohort might approach a billion.

With unicohorts ranging potentially from 1 to 100 million, it is convenient to compress them with the aid of base-10 logarithms to make the Safety-degree Scale[30], running from 0 to 8, as shown in Figure 10, which superimposes unicohort size on the corresponding units of the Safety-degree Scale. Note that the Scale avoids the semantic trap of absolute safety/zero risk by allowing safety-degree to rise without limit. Zero safety-degree corresponds to 1 in 1 certainty of adversity.

The Safety-degree Scale can be used to compare the risks posed by various hazards in life, as Figure 11 shows. Its use for medicines is illustrated by Figure 12, which shows how the risk of premature death from cardiovascular accidents in women taking high-dose oral contraceptives varies with age and smoking – data from the RCGP study[31]. Figure 13 shows how the overall safety-degree of life varies with age and sex, reflecting mortality from all causes.

Thus, the Safety-degree Scale is a convenient and simple format for communicating information about the probability of occurrence of adversity in life. The Safety-degree Scale reflects absolute risk and thus provides a way for people to compare risks posed by familiar and unfamiliar hazards to life. The Safety-degree Scale is not restricted merely to death, but is applicable to any stated adversity. The problem, of course,

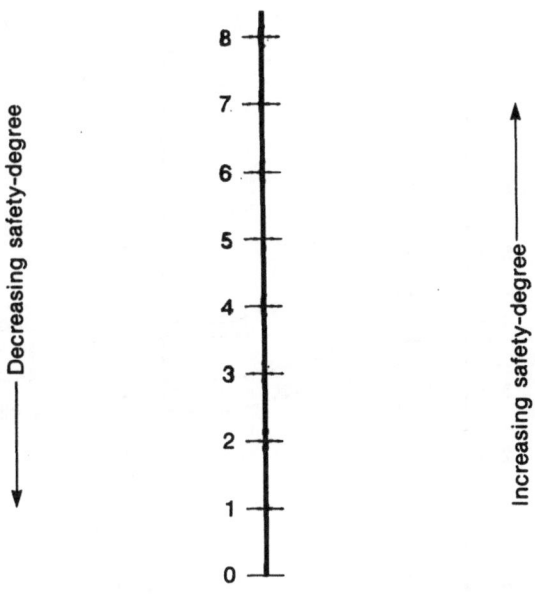

Figure 10 Schematic diagram of the Safety-degree Scale and the relation of its units to unicohort size

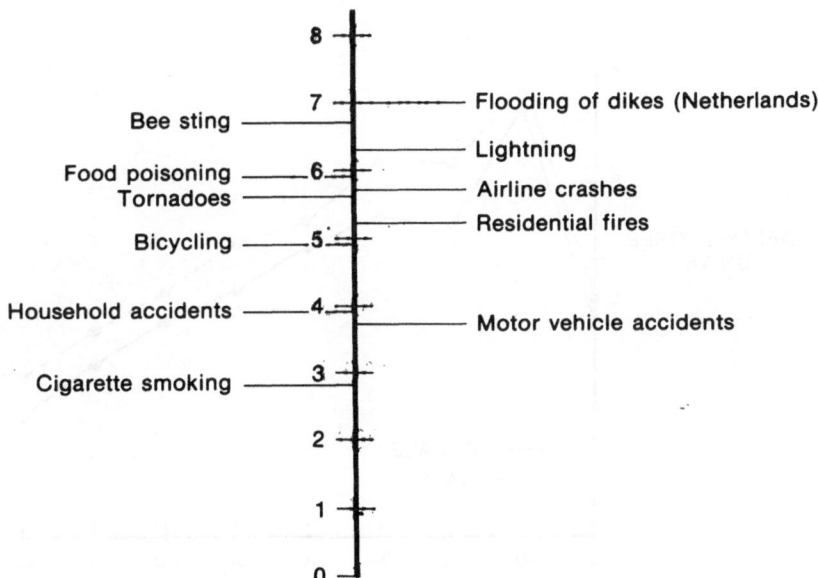

Figure 11 Degrees of safety of various of life's hazards. The sources of data for these safety-degree values can be found in Reference 32

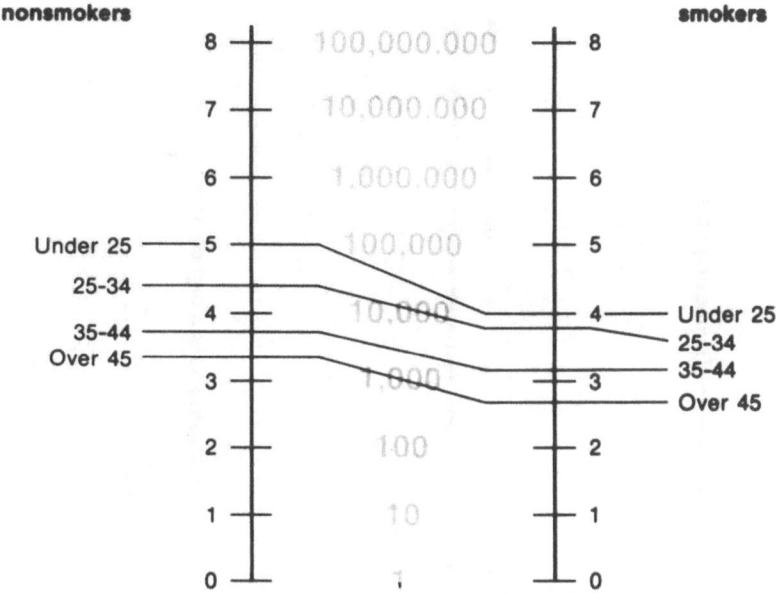

Figure 12 Age- and smoking-dependent safety-degree of using high dose oral contraceptive pills. The data are derived from the Royal College of General Practitioners' Study[31]

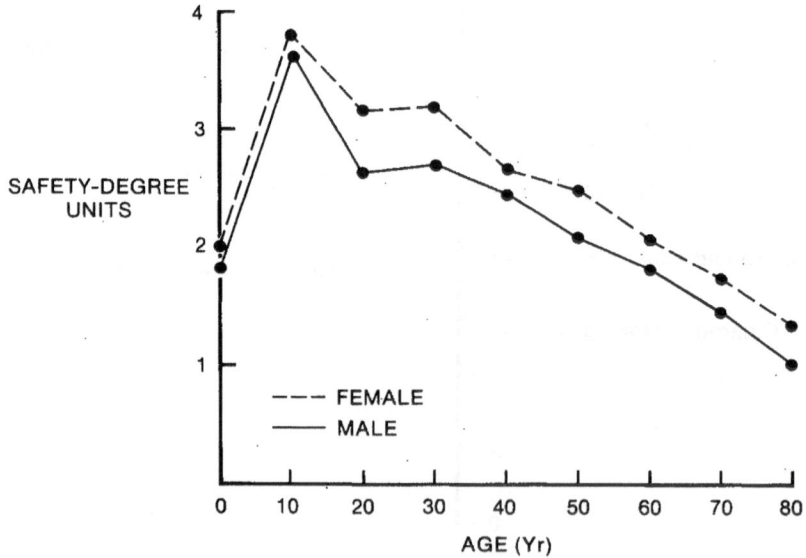

Figure 13 Age-dependence of the overall safety-degree of life. The data are computed from 1980 American mortality data[33]

with non-lethal endpoints, such as disabilities, is that data are sparse and the prospects for ameliorating that situation are entangled with serious issues of confidentiality. If such data become available, however, the Safety-degree Scale can serve as the means of communicating the probabilities of their occurrence.

DRUG 'SAFETY' vs DRUG SAFETY-DEGREE

The commonest problem in the testing of new drugs is to interpret the meaning of no observed adverse events, which one might conveniently refer to as the 'zero numerator' situation. Having zero in the numerator does not prove drug safety – it merely serves to estimate a degree of safety whose magnitude depends upon the number of patients and the time period over which observations were made. There are formal statistical considerations in interpreting the 'zero numerator'[34], notably, for studies involving more than 50 patients, the 'rule of three'[34]: if there are zero adverse events in n patient-years of treatment, one may have 95% confidence that the per-year risk of an adverse event is less than 1 in $n/3$. In the format of the Safety-degree Scale, one would say that the clinical trial has sufficed to define the per-year safety-degree of using the drug to a level of log $n/3$ SDU. An exceptionally large pre-market clinical trial, for example, might have as many as 2000 patients studied during one year of drug use; were there no observed adverse events, such pre-market experience would define the drug's per-year safety-degree as 2.8 SDU.

While a pre-market drug trial involving several thousand patients is quite large by current standards, it gives a very meagre definition of the safety-degree of drug use. That fact is illustrated by recent product withdrawals, accompanied by much public dismay, once the drug-related risk of serious or fatal adverse reactions turned out to be of the order of 1 in 5–10000 per treatment cycle – i.e. 3.7–4 SDU. While there is considerable softness in the available data, it would appear that the risk of life-threatening or fatal adverse reactions with tienilic acid, benoxaprofen, a long duration controlled release oral form of indomethacin, and indoprofen were of the order of 1 in 5–10000 per treatment cycle. The recent withdrawal of isoxicam from the French market appears to have been for a fatal adverse reaction occurring at the level of 1 in about 60 000 per treatment cycle (4.8 SDU). Thus, there is a discrepancy of 1–2 orders of magnitude between the degree of safety currently being defined by the largest pre-registration studies and the degree of safety that the public, its news media, and its politicians will accept for chronic or intermittent use in managing chronic diseases in ambulatory medicines.

One may note that the discrepancy may be further widened because it is sometimes inappropriate to use the entire patient population in clinical trials as the denominator for reckoning the estimate of drug safety-degree. If there are important considerations of sex, age, concomitant diseases, or concomitant treatments, then one has to consider the pre-registration trials results by subgroups, which necessarily reduces the defined safety-degree.

Few otherwise well-informed members of the public understand that only a relatively meagre degree of drug safety is definable before registration. Instead, the public believes that the long and costly process of regulation-mandated pre-market testing is providing drugs that are 'safe'. The big discrepancy between fact and expectation is part of the reason why the news media have periodic extravaganzas of shock and horror when serious adverse reactions first come to light. Unfortunately, these shock-horror episodes arouse strong feelings and demands for action, the politically easiest of which is to force product withdrawal. Generally, the preferable path would be restrictive relabelling, to preserve the product for those in whom its use is beneficial. However, that path usually closes when media and politicians lock step in the war dance to invoke quick remedial action so that such things never happen again. Meanwhile, the public, which lacks any recognized way to understand the comparative risks involved, shuns the drug as a form of rat poison, but continues to drive, drink, smoke, jaywalk and eat Eggs Benedict, forgets to take its blood pressure pills and performs other risky activities with impunity and few, if any, second thoughts.

There is clearly a need for reliable mechanisms for monitoring the consequences of therapeutic intervention after the product upon which it is based is registered and enters the medical market[35]. But the need is not only to generate data, it is to provide a context for interpreting the results of such information. That need brings us back to the lack of a publicly accepted and understood scale for safety degree and risk information that permits all of us – not just experts – to see the risk of a new hazard in the context of life's familiar hazards. Perhaps if really interpretable information on drug-related risks were widely available, we could simplify and streamline the pre-registration testing of new drugs, bring valuable new drugs into general use sooner, rather than later.

References

1. *Science' 85*, **6** (8), 1985
2. Louis Harris and Associates: (1980). *Risk in a Complex Society - A Marsh & McLennan Public Opinion Survey.* (New York: Marsh & McLennan).
3. Starr, C. (1972) Benefit-cost studies in socio-technical systems. In *Perspectives on Benefit-Risk Decision Making.* (Washington, DC: National Academy of Engineering).
4. Kletz, T.A. (1977). The risk equations – what risks should we run? *New Scient.*, **74**, 320--2
5. Lord Rothschild. (1978). *Risk - the Richard Dimbleby Lecture. The Listener*, 30 November
6. Heilmann, K. and Urquhart, J. (1983). *Keine Angst vor der Angst: Risiko-Element unseres*

Lebens und Motor des Fortschritts. (Munich: Kindler Verlag)

7. Urquhart, J. and Heilmann, K. (1984). *Risk Watch: The Odds of Life.* (New York; Facts on File Publications)
8. *Ibid*, p.14
9. WHO Scientific Group on the Epidemiology of Aging: The Uses of Epidemiology in the Study of the Elderly. World Health Organization Technical Report Series 706, Geneva, 1984.
10. Fries, J.F. (1980). Ageing, natural death and the compression of mortality. *N. Engl. J. Med.*, **303**, 130–5
11. Education and Examination Committee of the Society of Actuaries (1977). Part 10 (LB), Study notes, 10 LB–507–81, (Chicago)
12. Anonymous (1985). Update: Acquired Immunodeficiency Syndrome – United States. *MMWR*, **34**, 245
13. Anonymous. (1982). Death on the road. *Wall St. J.*, 14 April
14. Dicke, W. (1982). States heeding pleas to strengthen laws on drunk driving. *NY Times*, 16 April
15. Reference 7, p. 89
16. Baker, S.P. O'Neill, B. and Karts, R.S. (1984). *Injury Fact Book.* Fig. 16–1. (Lexington MA: Lexington Books)
17. *Ibid*, Fig. 17–21
18. *Ibid*, Fig. 18–24
19. Brackenridge, R.D.C. (1977). *Medical Selection of Life Risks.* (London; Undershaft Press)
20. Comfort, A. (1984). Alcohol as a social drug and health hazard. *Lancet*, **1**, 443–4
21. Sherlock, S. (ed.). (1982). *Alcohol and Disease. Br. Med. Bull.*, **38**
22. US Department of Health, Education and Welfare. (1964). *Smoking and Health.* PHS Publ. No. 1103 (Washington DC; US Government Printing Office)
23. Cowell, M.J. and Hirst, B.C. (1980). Mortality differences between smokers and nonsmokers. *Trans. Soc. Actuaries*, **32**, 1–29
24. Hayes, T.C. (1981). Insurance gain for the nonsmoker. *NY Times*, 11 April
25. Society of Actuaries. (1959). *Build and Blood Pressure Study.* (Chicago)
26. Royal Society. (1983). *Risk Assessment – Report of a Royal Society Study Group.* (London)
27. Sills, D.L. (1985). Hazards beyond number. *Nature*, **317**, 117–18
28. British Standards Institution. (1979). *Glossary of Terms Used in Quality Assurance (Including Reliability and Maintainability Terms).* BS 4778 (London).
29. US Congress, Office of Technology Assessment. (1978). *Assessing the Efficacy and Safety of Medical Technologies.* (Washington, DC)
30. Reference 7, pp. 47–51, 190–195
31. Royal College of General Practitioners, Oral Contraceptive Study. (1977). Mortality among oral contraceptive users. *Lancet*, **2**, 727–31
32. Reference 7, p. 49
33. US Bureau of the Census. (1980). *Statistical Abstract of the United States*, Table 108. (Washington, DC)
34. Hanley, J.A. and Lippman-Hand, A. (1983). If nothing goes wrong, is everything all right? *J. Am. Med. Assoc.*, 1743–5
35. Inman, W.H.W. (1985). Risks in Medical Intervention. In Cooper, M.G. (ed.). *Man-made Hazards to Man.* (Oxford: Clarendon)

Risks in Perspective

Discussion (Chairman: Professor A.W. Asscher)

CHAIRMAN: I would like to briefly summarize some of the points that may come up in discussion. Professor Lee told us a little about what makes people perceive risk in an odd, contorted way. He didn't actually touch on the role of the press, of politicians and perhaps of education in how the exaggerated perception of risk might be prevented. Professor Smith's account was interesting in relation to the entry and exit phenomenon in disease – are these uniformly distributed or should we have talked about high risk groups in relation to risk–benefit analysis of drug therapy? We ought perhaps to see how these groups can be identified if we are going to make an equation. Dr Urquhart dealt with the difficult task of quantification, and appeared to be veering towards money as the common denominator.

DR JONES: Professor Lee, when you ask the public to perceive risks and grade them, there are two elements. Firstly there is a rational element, whether they have knowledge. I have no idea of the risk of dying from hang-gliding compared with living near a nuclear power station. The second element is an emotional perception. Do you distinguish between these two elements in the perception of risk, because you may be able to do something about the first of them, i.e. you may be able to tell me what the mortality risk is from hang-gliding, whereas the second element is much more complicated? I would suggest that people may be mixing up benefit with their emotional reaction to risk.

PROFESSOR LEE: Although simplifications are sometimes useful, oversimplification can be dangerous and misleading. The evaluation that you make of hang-gliding, and you must be making an evaluation if you engage in it or don't engage in it, is complicated. It will include some knowledge of hang-gliding which is not quantitative but is comparative, i.e. you can't put a number to it but you probably know that it is similar to motorcycling and safer than vaccination. So you have some knowledge. You also associate the activity with a number of beliefs, that is that high status people engage in this kind of activity, and that it gives a feeling of emotional exhilaration and so on. So a complex evaluation, emotional and cognitive, clusters around hang-gliding.

43

That could obviously be changed, for example by direct experience or by an input from the press. In my view it cannot be changed by someone saying that the chances are 1 in a million. Simplification almost always means reducing it to mortality rates because of the power of bogus quantification in our society and because of the influence of the insurance industry. Ordinary people, in evaluating risks, are not too worried about quantitative mortality although policy makers may be and medical specialists should be. Don't forget, that whatever science does, it is usually the public that determines how much money is going to be spent. The public calls the tune, not scientists. So we do need to look very carefully at the public's evaluations which are more complex and in my opinion more influential.

DR URQUHART: I would like to make the point that perhaps the most expeditious way to find out the risk of hang-gliding is to watch what the insurance industry does to make special purpose insurance for hang-gliders. It is a 400-year-old industry, and it does a lot of special purpose pricing for the creation of policies. Therein hangs the beginning of quantification. If you look in the smoking literature, one of the strongest pieces of evidence for the adverse health consequences of smoking is the actuarial results from 20 years of history of offering premium discounts to non-smokers. As it has been published in the actuarial literature, most people in the medical world don't know about it. There is no-one here from the insurance industry, and their reticence to talk about this says something about how risk is perceived.

CHAIRMAN: The insurance business is pretty arbitrary, isn't it?

DR URQUHART: It is disciplined by a marketplace.

PROFESSOR RAWLINS: Richard Doll, I believe, demonstrated the early risk of smoking and the insurance business caught on to it. They didn't actually have the evidence that people were smoking when they took out their insurance.

PROFESSOR VERE: I feel that the effect of a single adverse experience, either in the life of an individual or of a culture, can form a perception of risk very markedly. In my first week as a medical student, I was asked to tell a patient that he had a bronchopleural fistula caused by lung cancer, so that he could settle his affairs. I explained the situation to the patient and his response was 'Oh, thank goodness for that. If you had told me it was TB I would have thrown myself out the window.' We subsequently discovered the reason for that response was that his father had died of tuberculosis. We have recently, as a medical school, had to renegotiate our insurance premium for clinical pharmacological studies. We found the insurance company obsessed by the thought of the deaths of two volunteers in this type of study relatively recently, despite the fact that neither of those deaths was necessarily related to the actual research process in hand in any way. They told us that it affected the market level. So a single adverse event has to be considered, and I don't know how our speakers would respond to that.

DR CROMIE: I would like to ask Dr Urquhart about his media-Richter scale. We have had this type of meeting with the press and they said that they never ask experts because they are always biased. I, therefore, wonder if there has been any progress in America of a media organization actually having one of these people trying to put risks into context.

DR URQUHART: No. I think that will probably happen in the Netherlands before it happens in the States. That is a much more manageable society and ideas are beginning to take root there.

DR FITZGERALD: Professor Lee, do we know when children begin to formulate the concept of risk? What do we know about changing attitudes to risk in relation to maturity?

PROFESSOR LEE: As early as 3, 4 or 5 years of age, I think. I am not familiar with this research area, but it has been most closely investigated in relation to children's perception of risk in relation to traffic accidents. That is where they are taught about risk, for obvious reasons.

DR FITZGERALD: With regard to accidents, do they conform because they are going to get shouted at or because they realize that it is a risk? I suggest it is the former rather than the latter.

PROFESSOR LEE: It is both. They get shouted at but they see the wisdom of it as soon as they experience a grazed knee or an accident causes them pain. The only area we have explored is children's perception of the risks of nuclear energy, which we do by eliciting drawings from them of nuclear power stations. The association, for example, with nuclear war, death or the military is developed very early indeed.

DR FITZGERALD: Our concerns are the failure of getting the perception right, and if we take children and teach them about nuclear power stations we understand very well the real risks there. How much of these risks are in fact conditioned by the current cohort of people and by the huge exposure in the amount of television they watch? Is the perception of risk in the next generation going to be less acceptable than it is at the present time?

CHAIRMAN: Should this be part of health education?

DR URQUHART: There is a group at the University of California, Berkeley, that focusses on curricular development in secondary schools. They have picked up this area and are working up curricular packages for 9–11-year-old students. They are trying to decide whether to use the logarithmic approach or to use something like the linear insurance premium scheme.

PROFESSOR LEE: I don't want to give the impression that the public is always wrong and the scientist is always right and that the public needs to be straightened out. I think that the public perceives different aspects of the risk, it evaluates them quite differently because it enters different, more intangible things into the equation. For example it puts morbidity in much more than mortality, as mortality is not that important to people. It is not a matter of correcting people; scientists need as much education as the public.

DR FITZGERALD: I think the concerns are the quality of the input.

PROFESSOR SMITH: Surely individuals take intuitive cost–benefit decisions. They assess the relativities. In the early 1950s my principal leisure pursuit was motor racing. I gave up smoking and then thought about whether it was wise to do so and to carry on motor racing. So I actually started smoking again!

PROFESSOR DOLLERY: Professor Lee, it seemed to me that you were giving a greater surface of reasonableness to the public's perception of risk than I easily feel. For example, why is it particularly in the latter part of this century that there is tremendous concern about ecology whereas the risks from environmental pollution were much greater during the equivalent period in the 19th century? Why has this emerged now? Perhaps the word 'logic' should not be used, but it may be permissible to use the word 'fashion'. It seems that there is an ecological fashion, and that it is quite possible that attention will swing to something different in 10–15 years.

PROFESSOR LEE: I agree. It is the same sort of process that characterizes the medical profession, that there are changing fads and fashions of that kind. To be more charitable, one could argue that the public has a sort of agenda, guided by charismatic figures that emerge and promote particular value systems at different times. As it has eliminated smallpox, tuberculosis and bubonic plague, and as it has established the technology that can give it relative wealth so that, in our civilisation it has abandoned hunger, it is coming around increasingly to what are called 'quality of life' variables. These are now seen to be intimately connected with the environment. The links between people and their environment, people and their food, people and their life-style are being seen as more and more important. It is almost patronizing to suggest that the public, of which we ourselves are members, are engaged in a capricious movement from one fad to another. On the other hand, the process is by no means random and certainly not logical in the conventional sense. People move their priorities in response to their changing needs and in response to stimulation they receive from leaders of society, including the medical profession.

Session 2

Assessing the Risks from Medicines

2.1 Risk predicted from animal studies

Professor G. Zbinden

CURRENT PRACTICE AND PROBLEMS

The concept that the first use of a new drug in man must always be preceded by safety studies in laboratory animals, and that additional toxicological experiments are performed before a marketing licence is requested, came into force almost 50 years ago. During this time, toxicological testing has developed into an enormously laborious effort, whose cost–effectiveness is now seriously disputed. Moreover, a third party, the drug regulatory agencies, is increasingly using safety and consumer protection as arguments to tighten its control over the drug development process. Therefore, it is understandable that medicinal chemists and pharmacologists on the one hand, and clinical pharmacologists on the other, regard pre-clinical safety investigations as a mixed blessing and, at best, as a costly insurance policy with limited coverage.

The problem of predictability of human risk from animal experiments is, of course, central to this debate. If hazardous compounds were reliably detected, and well tolerated drugs were consistently identified as agents presenting no relevant human risk, the heavy costs and the delays caused by toxicological testing programmes could be tolerated. Depending on one's position and temperament, the question whether or not current toxicological practice satisfies these requirements, is answered quite differently. In this presentation, the reasons for the diversity of opinions and the concepts which may be applied in predicting human risks from animal studies will be discussed.

A frequently encountered misconception makes a harmonious debate of these problems quite difficult: it is often not recognized that the primary purpose of a toxicological experiment is to know the whole spectrum of adverse characteristics of a drug. For this reason, one tries to detect as many toxic effects of a chemical as possible, and to determine their relationship to dose, time and route of administration and their occurrence in different animal species. In contrast, many outsiders look at toxicity data with nothing else in mind than human risk. They are happy when the tests are negative, and take most changes induced in animals as a sign of danger for the patients. As a consequence, they will often be frightened by toxic responses which later prove to be irrelevant to man, and almost as often they will be surprised by adverse reactions in humans which the animal models failed to demonstrate. Other experimental findings for which it is difficult to imagine a corresponding human disease, such as a positive Ames test, further add to the confusion.

Over the years, much information on adverse effects of many drugs in animals and man has accumulated. Some of the lessons learnt are discussed in this paper.

EXTRAPOLATION OF 'NEGATIVE' RESULTS

In most animal tests, only a few organs and organ systems are identified in which treatment-related toxic effects develop. But much effort is made to extrapolate these 'positive' findings to man, and to warn the clinicians to watch out even for the most remote possibility of injury. In contrast, if a test compound has not caused organ damage in animals, it is rare indeed that toxicologists worry about the meaning for man. But the same people then write indignant articles on the failure of toxicity studies to detect certain adverse effects such as anaphylactic shock, jaundice and hallucinations.

It is important to recognize that only some of the 'negative' toxicological findings in animal models are due to a lack of toxic properties. Many other reasons are listed in Table 7. Thus, before a compound which is well tolerated in animals can be considered safe for humans, one has to determine whether or not this prediction is justified. Unfortunately, the techniques to extrapolate 'negative' experimental data are not yet well developed. But this does not give one the right to forget about the problem altogether.

EXTRAPOLATION OF 'POSITIVE' RESULTS

A toxicological alert is usually sounded when adverse effects are identified in an animal model. The inference from almost any toxic response occurring in an animal test that patients taking the drug could be harmed, has already been deplored. The four important questions which need to be answered when one is faced with toxic responses in safety tests, will be discussed, and are listed in Table 8.

The first point, namely the question whether or not an effect observed

Table 7   Reasons for negative toxicological findings

Test substance is not toxic
Toxic concentration in target organ not reached
Toxic concentration in target organ reached for insufficient length of time
Insufficient sample size
Anatomical and physiological species differences
Use of unsuitable animal model
Development of tolerance
Toxic effects present but not detectable
Toxic effect present but not looked for

Table 8   Questions asked in the face of positive toxicological findings in animals

Is the effect real?
Is lesion likely to occur in man under comparable circumstances?
Is lesion likely to occur in man under realistic circumstances of use?
Are there special risk populations?

in animals is caused by the treatment, poses a particularly thorny problem. In all experimental sciences, the ability to reproduce a finding, is considered to be the decisive proof of validity. However, in toxicology, it is often impossible to repeat an experiment, because of the time and cost involved. In addition, even if a test is re-done, and the original result cannot be confirmed, the first observation remains on the books, and is considered at least as putative evidence of human risk. Thus, in such cases, the process of extrapolation of toxicological observation is burdened with a perplexing element of doubt.

When the toxic effects seen in animal tests are clearly treatment-related, it is often difficult to determine whether or not a corresponding adverse reaction is likely to occur in patients. Moreover, the available data-base often does not permit one to predict the critical dose, the special circumstances which might favour the development of a toxic reaction and the characteristics of risk populations.

Because of the limited information gained even with a comprehensive toxicological investigation, the process of extrapolation still derives much benefit from empirical data. The most important information is the cumulative knowledge obtained with older chemicals, with which toxicological studies were performed either before or after their introduction into the human environment. From this experience it is safe to assume that a toxic response which is dose- and time-related and which is demonstrable in several mammalian species, is also likely to develop in humans. Such predictions are particularly accurate, if one deals with compounds which are chemically and pharmacologically related to known reference drugs.

The knowledge that a compound is most probably hazardous to man is, of course, not sufficient to determine human risk. All it says is that the drug could induce the same lesions as in the animals, but whether or not it would do so under realistic conditions of use requires much additional information. For example, when Antopol and Tarlov in 1942 induced sensory neuropathy in dogs and rats with vitamin B6 using doses as high as 3 g/kg, the prediction was justified that comparable lesions would also occur in man[1]. However, at this time, the vitamin was used as a nutritional supplement in doses of less than 0.1 mg/kg, and the question of human risk was never even considered. Only much later, when vitamin megatherapy became fashionable, were daily doses of 2–6 g pyridoxin prescribed, and the development of sensory neuropathy in several patients proved that the original toxicological observation could indeed be extrapolated to man[2].

The example shows that the dose necessary to induce a toxic lesion is an important aspect in extrapolating animal toxicity data to man. As demonstrated in Table 9, the doses found to be toxic in laboratory animals are often surprisingly close to those causing comparable changes in human subjects. There are, of course, many exceptions, and often, the degree of correspondence differs much from one animal species to the other (e.g. paracetamol). From this observation it must be concluded that it is, in general, not the dose which decides the extent of the organ damage but the actual target organ exposure which is determined mainly by the product of organ concentration and time. Thus, it is not sufficient to know the toxic dose in animals and the therapeutic dose in humans, but the knowledge of the pharmacokinetic parameters in the various species is essential in order to arrive at a realistic risk estimate for man. For example, in order to produce ECG changes in rats with protriptyline, daily doses of 2 × 16–32 mg/kg were necessary. In order to predict whether or not similar changes would occur in humans with the therapeutic dose of approximately 0.7 mg/kg, it was necessary to determine plasma concentrations. It was found that the critical plasma levels causing identical ECG changes were of the same order of magnitude in rats and humans[3] (Table 10).

The examples of cyclosporin A and thalidomide (Table 9) illustrate the most serious difficulty in extrapolating animal safety data to man: it is the problem of those species differences which cannot be explained solely by variations of pharmacokinetic parameters. Experience shows that fundamental differences in response to chemicals in various species of laboratory animals are frequent, and in some cases, such differences also occur not only between species, but also between sexes. This is quite often

Table 9   Dose- and time-related toxic responses[a]

Substance	Toxic effect	Animal	Man
NP 207	retinopathy	cat 10–70[r]	3–40[r]
Furosemide	hypokalaemia	rat 50–100	3[r]
Doxorubicin	cardiomyopathy	rabbit 300–500[r]*	500[r]*
Cyclophosphamide	cystitis	rat 15[r]	1.5[r]
Gentamicin	nephrotoxicity	rat 5–40[r]	5+[r]
Trimanyl	phospholipidosis	rat 4[r]	2.5[r]
		monkey 6–12.5[r]	
Nitrofurantoin	testicular atrophy	rat 150[r]	10+[r]
Ethinyloestradiol	cystic endometrial	dog 0.01[r]	0.05–0.1[r]
	hyperplasia		
Thalidomide	phocomelia	*Macaca arcoides*	1.7[r]
		1.25[r]	
		rabbit 50–150[r]	
		rat[nte]	
Paracetamol	liver necrosis	mouse, hamster	215–430[s]
		250–375[s]	
		rat ca 1200–1500[s]	
Cyclosporin A	nephrotoxicity	rat 45[r]	ca 40[r]
		rhesus monkey 300[nte]	
		dog 45[nte]	

[a]   = Doses in mg/kg
r   = repeated dose
s   = single dose
nte = no toxic effect observed
*   = mg/m^2

All data from Zbinden[3a] (1985)

Table 10   ECG changes and serum concentrations of protriptyline in rats. Animals treated twice daily with doses ranging from 16 to 32 mg/kg p.o.

Effect	Minimum serum concentration, µg/l
Positive chronotropic effect	30
Prolongation of QRS interval	96–116
Increase of T wave voltage amplitude	45–96
Prolongation of PQ interval	528
Therapeutic serum concentrations in patients on 40 mg/day:	113–376

Zbinden *et al.*[3b] (1980)

seen in carcinogenicity studies where sex differences in tumour response are the rule rather than the exception.

It is often claimed that species differences are mainly due to differences in metabolism. While the hypothesis is supported by some classical examples (e.g. the high sensitivity of dogs against arylamines because of their inability to acetylate these compounds), it is common experience that fundamental differences in metabolism can rarely be identified as the major reasons for species differences in drug toxicology. Many other factors must play a role. For example, retinopathy due to phenothiazines occurs only in dogs and cats, but not in the albino rat, because binding to melanin in the chorioid is an essential prerequisite for the accumulation of the drugs at the target site[4].

RISK ASSESSMENT IN THE LIGHT OF SPECIES DIFFERENCES

Unfortunately, in most cases in which clear-cut species differences are detected in pre-clinical safety studies, it is not possible to identify the reasons. Under such circumstances, the prediction of the likely human response and the assessment of human risk are more a matter of judgement than a result of scientific argument. Some of the important factors which must be entered into the decision-making process are summarized in Table 11. The time-honoured safety factor (Table 12), still dear to the heart of many toxicologists, is used mainly for risk assessment of environmental chemicals. In drug toxicology, it is hardly acceptable to take the 'no adverse effect level' in the most sensitive species as the major determinant for human risk. Biomechanistic and pharmacokinetic con-

Table 11   Factors to be considered in assessing human risk

No adverse effect level and safety factor
Blood and tissue concentrations at toxic and therapeutic doses
Previous experience with related substances
Observations in different animal species
Cell type, tissue, organ and organ systems affected
Reversibility of lesion
'Seriousness' of lesion
Biological mechanism of toxic response
Availability of markers for patient monitoring

Table 12   Consideration of dose in assessment of human risk

Conduct toxicological animal studies
Determine most sensitive species
Determine no adverse effect dose
Apply safety factor to correct for species differences
Apply safety factor to correct for special risk populations
Calculate acceptable daily dose and determine human risk at proposed therapeutic dose

siderations coupled with insights from past experience must be combined to arrive at a realistic estimation of risk.

If the question of admissibility of clinical trials is raised, it becomes necessary to judge the nature of the toxic response seen in animal experiments. Some of the deciding factors, also listed in Table 11, can be investigated experimentally. Among these are the questions of reversibility of the lesions and the vital importance of the target cells. Also important is the availability of objective signs and markers which can be used to detect the existence of a toxic lesion and which can be used for patient monitoring. Finally, often an estimate of the therapeutic benefit also creeps into the risk assessment process, although, strictly speaking, it should be dealt with on a different level.

CONCLUSIONS

The assessment of human risk of a new drug is a multi-stage process. It begins with the collection of toxicological data and their assembly in a toxicological dossier. Unfortunately, predictions of human risk, and decisions about the future fate of the test substance are often made before many other essential steps are undertaken. Particularly important is the acquisition of knowledge of pharmacokinetic characteristics of the drug and its metabolism in laboratory animals and in man.

The evaluation of the toxicological data must consider two empirical facts: (1) toxic changes observed in animal experiments also frequently occur in man, and (2) sometimes the responses in animals and man are different. The reasons are either special circumstances of use (e.g. overdosage) or differences in structure and function of the organs or diversities of drug metabolism. The first fact reminds us to treat toxicological studies with respect. The second fact warns us that the extrapolation of toxicological results, be they 'positive' or 'negative', must be done with great care, and with due consideration of all biological characteristics of the toxicological models.

Once the evaluation process is completed and the extrapolation of the animal findings to man is made, an assessment of human risk can be attempted. For this, detailed knowledge of the characteristics of the exposed population (age, sex, disease state, etc.) must be available. The doses used in therapy, the resulting blood and tissue concentrations of the drug and its metabolites, and the routes and extent of elimination must be considered. If marked species and sex differences are uncovered in the pre-clinical safety studies, the assessment of human risk becomes very critical. Unless the reasons for such differences can be elucidated, risk assessment becomes mainly a matter of judgement, and the ultimate burden of proof of safety must be left with the clinical investigator.

References

1.   Antopol, W. and Tarlov, I.M. (1942). Experimental study of the effects produced by large doses of vitamin B6. *J. Neuropath. Exp. Neurol.*, **1**, 330–6

2.   Schaumburg, H.H., Kaplan, J., Windebank, A., Vick, N., Rasmus, S., Pleasure, D., and Brown, M.J. (1983). Sensory neuropathy from pyridoxin abuse. A new megavitamin syndrome. *N. Engl. J. Med.*, **309**, 445–8

3(a). Zbinden, G. (1985). *Menschen, Tiere und Chemie.* (Zollikon: MTC Verlag)

3(b). Zbinden, G., Ettlin, R. and Bachmann, E. (1980). Electrocardiographic changes in rats during chronic treatment with antidepressant and neuroleptic drugs. *Arzneimittel Forsch.*, **10**, 1709–15

4.   Meier-Ruge, W. (1967). *Medikamentöse Retinopathie.* (Stuttgart: Georg Thieme Verlag)

2.2 The risk identified from clinical trials

Professor C.T. Dollery

Toxicology is not a black art but a science which belongs to the general group of the pharmacological sciences. As such it must be analysed in terms of factors such as dose, route of administration, duration of exposure and individual (usually genetic) predisposition. The reason that toxicology, both in animals and in man, often does appear to be more of an art than a science is that prescribers, regulators and industrialists usually have to make their decisions on the basis of inadequate data. They do so in the name, often quite reasonably, of trying to minimize risk.

My charge is to discuss clinical trials, by which I mean deliberate, formal experiments in man where a number of individuals are exposed to the same closely specified protocol. It is usual to use the terminology devised by the Federal Drug Administration, and to divide clinical trials into stages. Each stage has a different objective, as shown in Table 13.

Stage 1 is tolerance and dose-ranging, and the total experience in patient years is usually less than 1 since often only single doses are given. The objective of stage 2 is pharmacokinetics, including metabolism, plasma concentration, etc, and early studies of pharmacodynamics, i.e. the mechanism of action of the drug in man. The total of these is often less

Table 13   Stages of clinical trials

Stage	Objective	Total patient years exposure
1	Tolerance, Dose-ranging	<1
2	Pharmocokinetics Pharmacodynamics	<5
3	Efficacy	<500
4	Monitoring (PMS)	<10000
	Outcome	<100000

than 5 patient years, because typically such studies are only single-doses or perhaps up to 2 weeks exposure. Stage 3 is, broadly speaking, efficacy studies. This is usually efficacy in a pharmacological sense, for example does the drug consistently lower blood pressure or control blood sugar. It is not an outcome trial and is not usually answering the question, 'Does this drug benefit patients with hypertension or diabetes?'. It is at this stage that drugs are brought to a licensing authority for marketing. The total exposure is usually less than 500 patient years at that time, because typically there will be 1–3000 patients treated mostly for short periods, usually 6 weeks and only 100 for as long as a year. The fourth stage is the monitoring stage, usually less than 10000 patient years, and Professor Lawson will be talking about this. I would like to devote most of my talk to outcome trials. These may be very large and may approach 100000 patient years. If you bear in mind that it is not possible to make a decision based on a single incident of any particular event, unless it is highly unusual, you can see that the sensitivity of any of these studies is not very high.

It is difficult to make generalizations about the value of these trials, certainly in a scientific sense, because each trial and each drug is different. I think it would be fair to say that toxicology has proved to be reasonably effective in preventing the introduction of compounds with high and unknown toxicity into clinical trials. Many drugs with high toxicity, such as doxorubicin and cyclophosphamide, have been introduced into clinical trials, but generally their toxicity had been fairly well predicted by animal studies. There are, however, two areas where the predictions are relatively poor:

(1)   It is not very easy to detect CNS effects in animals that may cause very unpleasant symptoms in man, although they are very unlikely to be lethal, for example dizziness, vertigo, convulsions. In my own experience of unpleasant events during early drug studies CNS symptoms, sometimes quite severe, figure highly.

(2)   There are no practical models in animal studies for toxic effects that have an immunological mechanism, for example Stevens–Johnson syndrome and drug-induced lupus.

However, these are not the most common problems that I see as a conductor of clinical trials, as an evaluator (being a past member of the Committee on Safety of Medicines) and as an occasional consultant to the pharmaceutical industry. The most common problem occurs when a patient on an investigational drug falls ill, for example they become jaundiced or are found to have neutropenia. It is then difficult to decide whether the drug is responsible, or whether the effect is due to intercurrent diseases. Thorough investigation and documentation of such morbid events does help. These events are a medical emergency, not for the patient, but for the drug and the community. There may, therefore, be a conflict in that you may seriously wish to do a liver biopsy or a bone marrow examination which is not, strictly speaking, clinically indicated or necessary for patient management, but is very important in coming to a decision regarding the cause of the event. Benefit and risk decisions at that stage often have to be made with incomplete data of variable quality, with inadequate knowledge of the incidence and very limited information about potential benefits.

The only situation where there is a reasonable balance sheet is when a large scale outcome trial has been carried out. It might be thought, following on from what I have said, that if one has sufficient data to give reasonably reliable information about all the benefits and risks, that it would make life a lot easier. I would now like to examine this proposition, as I would suggest that this is not necessarily so.

Clinical trials used to be conducted largely to determine efficacy, but the large-scale outcome trial is at least as valuable as a determinant of accurate information about toxicity. Three examples of which are the University Group Diabetes Project (UGDP), the WHO clofibrate trial and the MRC Hypertension trial. The UGDP was a study conducted about 10 years ago in the United States, comparing different regimes for the treatment of diabetes – diet, insulin and various oral hypoglycaemics. The results strongly suggested that the oral hypoglycaemics increased the risk of myocardial infarction. The trial design was heavily criticized, but on the whole any flaws in its design were not sufficient to invalidate the conclusion, yet it has had relatively little influence on the treatment of diabetes. Admittedly, the drugs used now are different, but they have very closely related chemical structures and similar pharmacodynamic action to earlier oral hypoglycaemics. So the availability of this information seems to have had little influence.

The WHO clofibrate trial[1] was a randomized controlled trial comparing the value of clofibrate in the primary prevention of myocardial infarction. It was carried out in groups of people drawn from population samples who had cholesterol levels in the upper half of the normal range. The high cholesterol control group would be expected to have a similar mortality and morbidity experience to the clofibrate-treated groups. However, as shown in Table 14 there was a statistically significant excess of deaths in the clofibrate-treated group. There was not, as was hoped, a reduction in deaths from ischaemic heart disease, although there was a reduction in non-fatal myocardial infarction. The increased incidence of cholecystectomy was predicted. There has been a great deal of argument as to whether this finding is real, but I think the evidence suggests it probably is. The difficulty is that the increase in mortality does not really occur in any particular category, even within the increase in malignant neoplasms which were mainly of the gastro-intestinal tract but not of any

Table 14 Deaths in the trial and within 1 year of leaving it. Main cause groups. Numbers of deaths and rates at ages 30–59, and age-standardized rates per 1000 per annum at ages 40–59.

Cause of death	Group I			Group II			Group III		
	Clofibrate			High cholesterol control			Low cholesterol control		
	No. (All Ages)	Rate	St. Rate 40–59	No. (All Ages)	Rate	St. Rate 40–59	No. (All Ages)	Rate	St. Rate 40–59
Ischaemic heart disease	54	1.6	2.1	48	1.4	2.1	20	0.6	0.8
Other vascular	14	0.4	0.5	14	0.4	0.6	9	0.3	0.5
Neoplasm: malignant	58	1.7	2.2	42	1.3	1.7	41	1.3	2.5
Neoplasm: benign	3	—	—	—	—	—	1	—	—
Other medical causes	16*	0.5*	0.8*	5*	0.2*	0.2*	7	0.2	0.4
Accidents and violence	17	0.5	0.6	18	0.5	0.6	15	0.5	0.6
All causes other than IHD	108*	3.2*	4.1	79*	2.4*	3.1	73	2.3	3.9
All causes other than IHD, vascular and accidents and violence	77**	2.3**	3.1*	47**	1.4**	1.9*	49	1.5	2.9
Total all causes	162*	4.9*	6.2	127*	3.8*	5.2	93	2.9	4.7

*Significant difference between Groups 1 and II ($p < 0.05$)
**Significant difference between Groups 1 and II ($p < 0.01$)

particular pathological sort. So the evidence from this suggests firstly that the drug is not effective for its primary purpose, and secondly that it may be increasing overall mortality. Clofibrate was virtually withdrawn from use in most countries of the world, but the use of very closely related drugs such as bezafibrate, which have not been subjected to this particular analytical tool, has been expanding rapidly. If the observed effects of clofibrate are true, then it is quite likely that they also apply to a related drug like bezafibrate.

My final point, the problem of weighing unlike quantities, is illustrated by the MRC hypertension trial[2]. It was a large trial with about 18 000 patients who were studied for a period of 5 years. They were randomly allocated to one of two treatment regimes, either bendrofluazide or propranolol, or to matching placebos. Many observations were made during the trial, illustrating that a great deal of useful information can be obtained by 'bolting on' the side of a large outcome trial. Routine ECGs were carried out, and an increased frequency of ventricular ectopic beats was noted in the bendrofluazide-treated group.

One of the most useful pieces of information collected was the reasons why people on the trial had been withdrawn from a particular drug. In this context it is more useful to discover why people stopped a drug than to find out what happened to those who continued to take it. Quite unexpectedly, men on bendrafluazide were withdrawn at a reasonably high rate, about 1.7% per year, because of erectile impotence. There was also an increased incidence with propranolol, although considerably lower, as shown in Table 15. This shows that rather vague symptoms, which many would think are perhaps not drug-related, may indeed be. There was a substantial incidence of withdrawals due to nausea, dizziness and headache, particularly in women, in both the actively treated groups. There were substantial numbers of toxic effects leading to withdrawal, with an incidence of approximately 0.5–1% per patient per year.

The benefits in the trial are summarized in Table 16. The placebo rate for stroke was 2.6 per 1000 patient years, on propranolol it was 1.9 and on bendrafluazide it was 0.8. That is, in many ways, a remarkable degree of efficacy because it is a reduction by two thirds in the incidence of stroke. There are not many treatments as effective as that for any disease. On the other hand, there was no clear trend with coronary events, and there is no difference in total deaths. This is shown in more detail in Figure 14. Bendrafluazide is quite effective in markedly reducing placebo events in both smokers and non-smokers. Propranolol, however, is only effective in non-smokers and is completely ineffective in smokers. As far as I know, there was no suspicion of this great difference before this trial. There was some evidence that blood pressure control was slightly less effective with propranolol in smokers than non-smokers, which was true in this trial. Although propranolol did reduce the blood pressure in smokers it did not prevent stroke. Similarly, if one looks at all cardiovascular events as shown in Figure 14, it can be seen that events are lower in non-smokers throughout and that there is a hint that propranolol may reduce events, but this only was significant in non-smoking men.

One of the most difficult analyses is that of all causes of mortality by sex rather than treatment regime, as shown in Table 17. In men the mortality was a little lower in the actively treated group (10–15% less), whereas in the women it was about 20% higher. Neither of the individual sex comparisons with their matching placebos is statistically significantly different. However, taking all the data into account, with an interaction analysis there is a statistical difference between men and women. Therefore, when treated there is a trend that women show an increased mortality in contrast to men.

Randomized controlled trials of the large-scale outcome type do have an immense advantage in that there is a complete record of events, thus an increased incidence of common disease may be detected. On the other hand they have the disadvantage that large numbers are required for long periods of time and they are expensive. However, the real problem is that of weighing up unlike quantities. Within the MRC trial there is good evidence that treatment, particularly bendrafluazide, reduces stroke. On the other hand, there is also reasonably good evidence that, at least in women, mortality may be increased by treatment. One of the epidemiolo-

Table 15 Principal reasons for withdrawal from randomized treatment. Numbers of reports and rates/1000 patient years†
(Reproduced from *British Medical Journal* by permission of the authors and the Editor)

	Men						Women					
	Bendrofluazide		Propranolol		Placebos		Bendrofluazide		Propranolol		Placebos	
	No	Rate	No	Rate	No	Rate	No	Rate	No	Rate	No	Rate
Impaired glucose tolerance	60	7.7***	27	3.4	53	3.3	46	5.9***	16	2.1	31	2.0
Gout‡	100	12.8***	12	1.5	14	0.9	12	1.5***	0		0	
Impotence	96	12.6***	50	6.3***	20	1.3	0		0		0	
Raynaud's phenomenon	0		41	5.1***	3	0.2	2	0.3	34	4.5***	4	0.3
Skin disorder	6	0.8	12	1.5**	5	0.3	3	0.4	9	1.2**	2	0.1
Dyspnoea	1	0.1	57	7.1***	7	0.4	2	0.3	53	7.1***	3	0.2
Lethargy	28	3.6***	42	5.3***	8	0.5	13	1.7***	62	8.3***	4	0.3
Nausea, dizziness, or headache	33	4.2***	33	4.1***	22	1.4	58	7.4***	70	9.4***	27	1.8
Pressure at or above levels requiring change of treatment	8	1.0***	33	4.1***	611	38.2	11	1.4***	24	3.2***	400	26.0

† Patient years of observation relates here only to years accrued before withdrawal of randomized treatment.
‡ Defined as symptoms plus serum urate values in excess of 500 μmol/l in men, 450 μmol/l in women.
** $p < 0.01$; *** $p < 0.001$; p values are for comparison of rate on individual active drug with rate on placebos.

Table 16 Principal events by randomly allocated drug, both sexes together*
(Reproduced from British Medical Journal by permission of the authors and Editor)

	Bendrofluazide		Propranolol		Placebos		% Difference		Absolute difference/1000 patient years	
	No	Rate	No	Rate	No	Rate	Bendrofluazide	Propranolol	Bendrofluazide	Propranolol
Strokes	18	0.8	42	1.9	109	2.6	67	24	1.7	0.6
Coronary events	119	5.6	103	4.8	234	5.5	-2	13	-0.1	0.7
All cardiovascular events	140	6.6	146	6.7	352	8.2	20	18	1.7	1.5
Non-cardiovascular deaths	59	2.8	55	2.5	114	2.7	-4	5	-0.1	0.1
All deaths	128	6.0	120	5.5	253	5.9	-2	6	-0.1	0.4

* Apparent discrepancies are due to rounding in the figures presented for the rates

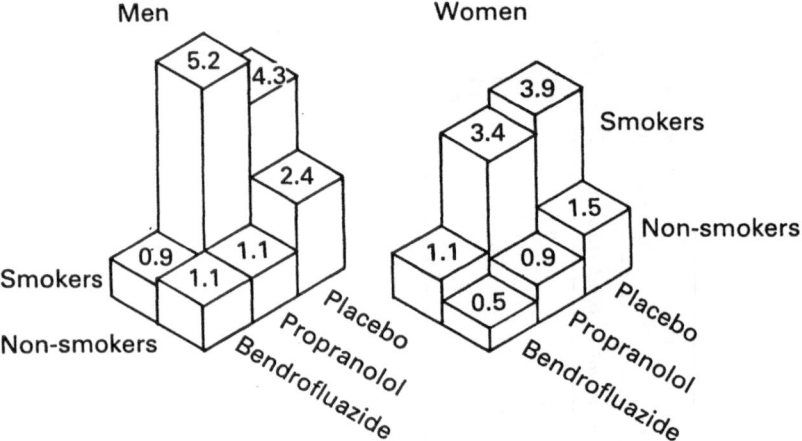

Figure 14 Incidence of stroke per 1000 person years of observation according to randomized treatment regimen and cigarette smoking status at entry to trial.

Table 17 Principal events by sex

	Active treatment		Placebo treatment		% Difference	Absolute difference/ 1000 patient year
	No	Rate	No	Rate		
Men						
Strokes	37	1.7	65	2.9	43	1.3
Coronary events	184	8.3	200	9.0	8	0.7
All cardiovascular events	225	10.2	272	12.3	17	2.1
Non-cardiovascular deaths	53	2.4	69	3.1	23	0.7
All deaths	157	7.1	181	8.2	13	1.1
Women						
Strokes	23	1.1	44	2.1	48	1.0
Coronary events	38	1.8	34	1.7	−11	−0.2
All cardiovascular events	61	2.9	80	3.9	25	1.0
Non-cardiovascular deaths	61	2.9	45	2.2	−34	−0.8
All deaths	91	4.4	72	3.5	−25	−0.9

gists associated with the MRC trial suggested that no-one with hypertension in this range should be treated, because of the results of the trial. However he found, to his surprise, that his patients' reaction was that they put more value on a reduction in stroke rather than the hazard of a small increase in mortality. At the end of the day with the trial, we have a reduction in stroke and some indication in one sub-group of a reduced mortality from myocardial infarction, while on the other hand there is a clear hint that overall mortality is increased in women and that there is a fairly high incidence of gout, diabetes, nausea, dizziness, impotence and so on. With all that information, it is still very difficult to make a sensible recommendations about treatment policy.

References

1. (1978). *Br. Heart J.* **40**, 1069–18
2. (1985). *Br. Med. J.* MRC trial of treatment of mild hypertension: principal result. Medical Research Council Working Party. **291,** 97–97

importance and so on. With an end like this, it will be very difficult to make a sensible recommendations about treatment etc.

References

2.3 The risk determined from PMS studies

Professor D.H. Lawson

In animal studies or in controlled clinical trials, investigators are looking for common beneficial or adverse outcomes. With these studies there is a relatively small number of factors which are likely to change at any one time. Mostly these are known and can be measured. Moreover, in most instances the time scales between first exposure and termination of the experiment are short, thus minimizing the period during which intervening variables can exercise a major effect on the study outcome. Indeed when we look at examples of trials in which there is a long delay between entry and end-point, we often find ourselves in areas of major controversy as regards the interpretations of the data – a situation not entirely dissimilar to that pertaining to most observational studies to date.

However, when we come to discuss post-marketing surveillance studies, we are venturing away from this relatively controlled area into one of uncontrolled observations with all the attendant difficulties that can arise from this.

Post-marketing surveillance is a term which means different things to different people. It can include the following diverse methodologies:

(1) The Yellow Card spontaneous reporting scheme in UK, and the unstructured types of case reports seen in journals. These usually function as alerting schemes, and as such make no pretence at estimating risk – being content merely to raise the possibility of there being a risk of condition X arising from the use of drug Y.

(2) The formal case-control study set up to test a specific hypothesis. This approach usually estimates relative risk rather than absolute risk or excess incidence; these latter parameters being only possible to measure where the case-control comparison is undertaken within the framework of a defined population.

(3) The type of observational cohort study undertaken by Professor Inman and his group in Southampton, by various manufacturers

including Sandoz (ketotifen), Reckitt and Colman (buprenor-phine) and Squibb (captopril), and by *ad hoc* groups such as Duncan Colin-Jones' group who looked at cimetidine recipients.

For the purposes of my discussion today, I wish to confine my remarks to the latter methodologies, partly because of time constraints and partly because of topical interest arising out of the increased pressure being brought to bear on industry to undertake such studies.

Although I see this objective of collecting more information, par-ticularly on newly released drugs, as very desirable, there are many potential pitfalls for the unwary investigator before these studies can produce information which will give an estimate of the risks to the patient arising from the use of the medicine(s) under study.

Patients, or should I say people, face a variety of hazards each day. These include such things as:

(1) Accidents or unexpected sudden illness;
(2) Consequences of previously unknown diseases – e.g. coronary or cerebral atherosclerosis (which may present as sudden death);
(3) Consequences of known diseases such as bronchitis, varicose veins, diabetes, etc;
(4) Sequelae of treated diseases such as cancer, epilepsy, glaucoma, psoriasis; and
(5) Finally complications of the drugs used to treat diseases or derived from symptoms with which the patient might present.

In PMS studies in which a cohort of patients are enrolled who are characterized by having received a specific medicine at one point in time, and are thereafter followed for an interval with the prime objective of determining the 'outcome' of that drug use, we have a variety of possible outcomes to consider (Figure 15).

(1) Patient develops a drug-induced disease – the 'risk' we are trying to measure;
(2) Patient develops a complication of the disease which caused the initial use of the drug;
(3) Patient develops a problem which cannot be determined whether it is drug-related or a complication or correlate of the indication for the drug;
(4) Patient expresses a manifestation of a previously diagnosed disease;
(5) Patient develops a new disease;
(6) Recurrent attendance for medical attention for disease A brings to light disease B;
(7) Patient develops a complication from use of another medicine.

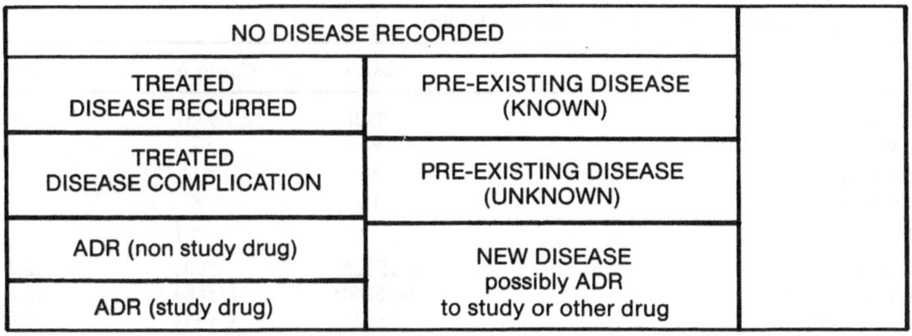

NO DISEASE RECORDED		
TREATED DISEASE RECURRED	PRE-EXISTING DISEASE (KNOWN)	
TREATED DISEASE COMPLICATION	PRE-EXISTING DISEASE (UNKNOWN)	
ADR (non study drug)	NEW DISEASE possibly ADR to study or other drug	
ADR (study drug)		

Figure 15 Outcomes in PMS studies

Diagrammatic representation of distribution of possible outcomes in an observational cohort study carried out over a substantial time period – say 1 year. ADR = Adverse Drug Reaction. Relative size of various compartments will vary according to type of drug studied and nature of underlying disease

You may think that these outcomes are theoretical rather than practical. I should however like to disabuse you of this thought by looking at examples from a study Duncan Colin-Jones, Michael Langman, Martin Vessey and I undertook at the request of Smith, Kline and French. This was a major PMS study of cimetidine. Details of the methods are published in the literature[1-3].

There are several points I wish to emphasize. Firstly, we had a comparator group of a sample of the population. The 'ideal' comparator of dyspeptic subjects not receiving cimetidine was impossible to attain when we started in 1976. Secondly, we compared disease frequencies in takers and controls over a 1 year period, and thereafter followed mortality in the taker group for many years. We have limited information on exposure status of recipients (numbers of prescriptions) because of the expense of collecting this information. We have no data on certain habits, e.g. smoking, alcohol, caffeine intake again because of expense constraints. We have 98% follow-up of the taker group at 1 year so missing details of patients who were drop-outs from the study was not a major problem in interpreting the results.

I should like now to point to some interesting results of our study (Table 18). In a 1 year follow-up we recorded 15325 diagnoses in takers and 5002 in the comparison group, i.e. many more 'events' in takers who were, therefore, a sicker group of patients. Thus a comparison of the two groups to determine an 'excess incidence' or risk is not really valid for many conditions. We detected a complication of the therapy – gynaecomastia which showed a 20-fold increase not 'expected' from the control group. We detected complications of the underlying disease – pancreatitis/perforation, cirrhosis, etc. We detected problems of previous

Table 18   Cimetidine PMS study – selected results

	Takers	Controls	RR
Number	9928	9351	1.0
1 year follow-up (%)	98.8	97.7	
OP visits (%)	39	21	
IP visits	18	8	
Death	3.7	2.1	
Diagnoses	15325	5002	3.2
Gynaecomastia	20/6240*	1/5884	18.8
Pancreatitis	10/9928	4/9351	2.6
Angina	38	19	2.1
Stroke	45	40	1.2
Cataracts	42	30	1.5
Cataracts removed	11	10	1.1
Rheumatoid arthritis	57	21	2.9
Lymphoma	32	10	3.4
Lung cancer	46	24	2.0
Chronic bronchitis	38	19	2.1
Asthma	25	23	1.2
Alcoholism	25	9	2.9

*6240 = number of male cimetidine takers
 5884 = number of male controls
 RR   = risk ratio

diseases such as hypertension, angina and strokes. We saw 'excess' frequencies of diagnoses coming to light as a result of increased physician contact, e.g. cataracts. We saw 'excess' frequencies of rheumatoid arthritis and of reticulosis – due to cimetidine being used to treat complications arising from the use of other drugs. We saw excess lung cancer – cimetidine identifying ulcer patients who have excess risk due to smoking and so of developing lung cancer and other smoking-related diseases. We also saw complications of other therapy, etc.

Thus in this study we found that we were unable truly to estimate global excess risks of cimetidine therapy as it was used in real life – which was our principal aim. However, we were able to reassure ourselves that cimetidine was not associated with a dramatic increase in an otherwise rare condition such as aplastic anaemia (a particular concern in view of the experiences of metiamide). Such negative information is often very useful and reassuring.

Future studies of this type will, I hope, concentrate on looking at restricted cohorts, e.g. of the elderly, the pregnant, those with renal failure, etc, thereby increasing their value by looking at those groups who have, in the past, been shown to be at special risk of developing drug-related problems.

Some problems can arise which are difficult to disentangle by using observational studies. Witness the continuing controversy over whether the undoubted association between the use of the anticonvulsant phenytoin and foetal malformations is due to the drug *per se* or due to epilepsy (or both). This is a very different topic to disentangle, since other anti-convulsants have also been reported to cause rather non-specific foetal malformations, and phenytoin itself is used for no other indication. Under such circumstances we may talk about the hazards faced by pregnant phenytoin recipients and quantify these by observational studies, but we may not know whether these hazards are truly risks of the drug itself or inherent risks of its indication.

In both these instances, we have examples of a major confounding variable causing problems in the interpretation of our data, that of the prime indication(s) for the study drug. This is a problem which is best solved by a controlled trial with randomized allocation to different treatment groups. Uncontrolled cohorts really only permit observations about diseases which are completely independent of the indication for starting the treatment.

If I can summarize, current technologies render PMS studies (cohort studies) feasible and practical, if one is thinking in terms of following 10–20000 people over relatively short periods of 1–5 years. Reasonable end-points can be achieved and interpreted. However, there are many pitfalls to avoid before even a suggestion of any new drug-induced problem can be made. In an ideal world – for the methodologist that is – drug-induced disease would be recognizably different from naturally occurring disease and would be easy to diagnose. In the real world, life is not so simple. In my view, we are at the same stage with PMS cohort studies now as we were with clinical trials in the early 1950s. Let us hope that we experience a similar learning curve to our more experimentally-minded colleagues over an equally short time interval. If we do, then by the mid–late 1990s we will know how to avoid the many pitfalls of PMS studies, and achieve a better ·new tool for assessing drug risks as they occur in the populations who actually take our medicines, rather than in the more idealized groups we would like to see taking them.

References

1. Colin-Jones, D.G., Langman, M.J.S., Vessey, M.P. and Lawson, D.H. (1982). Cimetidine and gastric cancer: preliminary report from post-marketing surveillance study. *Br. Med. J.*, **285**, 1311
2. Colin-Jones, D.G., Langman, M.J.S., Vessey, M.P. and Lawson, D.H. (1983). Post-marketing surveillance of the safety of cimetidine: 12 month mortality report. *Br. Med. J.*, **286**, 1713
3. Colin-Jones, D.G., Langman, M.J.S., Vessey, M.P. and Lawson, D.H. Post-marketing surveillance of the safety of cimetidine: 12 month morbidity report. *Q.J. Med.*, **54**, 215–253

Assessing the Risks from Medicines

Discussion (Chairman: Professor A.W. Asscher)

CHAIRMAN: We have had three contemplative and critical papers, somewhat self-effacing to some extent. Professor Zbinden made a good case for the value of animal studies, but of course there is no information on the drugs that are so toxic they never get into man. This is one of the major weaknesses of animal studies to which he did not make reference. Professor Dollery had great difficulty weighing up all the contradictory results from having almost too much information from the hypertension trials. The problem arose of the clinician having the difficulty of applying statistics to the individual patient. Professor Lawson was very critical of post-marketing surveillance studies. Professor Inman, would you like to make some comments?

PROFESSOR INMAN: The Lawson/Jones study took several years; the 1 year mortality data were published at the same time as the results of an 11 week PEM study of ranitidine. Remarkably, the data from the two studies, which were the same size but used completely different methods, were virtually identical.

Dr Urquhart in discussing the risk scale has a slightly different approach to mine because he chose to base his on the number of zeros. I have based my scale on the total number of digits, so we are an order of magnitude different. On our scale (Figure 16), the risk of contracting a disease is small compared with the risk associated with the disease itself. For example, the risk of tetanus is minute in the general population but once you have the disease the risk of dying is fairly enormous. Even a disease like rheumatoid arthritis is fairly dangerous.

Two questions that we may want to ask at some stage in this meeting are: (1) Why are drugs being removed from the market because of risks of death, when this risk is 100 or even 1000 times less than the risk of the disease? (2) What is an acceptable level of risk?

CHAIRMAN: Surely there will not be a standard figure for the acceptable level of risk – it will depend on the disease being treated.

Figure 16 Risk of death from certain diseases England and Wales, 1981 reproduced from Cooper, M.G. (1985). *Risk–Man-made Hazards to Man,* Oxford University Press, with permission

Risk level	Range (per year)	Cause of death
1	1 in 1– 9	
2	1 in 10–99	(Any cause)
3	1 in 100–999	Cancer, coronary disease, stroke
4	1 in 1 000–9 999	Peptic ulcer
5	1 in 10 000–99 999	Arthritis, asthma, cirrhosis, diabetes
6	1 in 100 000–999 999	Pregnancy*, VD
7	1 in 1 000 000–9 999 999	Tetanus, measles, whooping cough
8	1 in 10 000 000–99 999 999	Acute rheumatic fever

*Females only

Comparison of annual death rate in general population and in groups of patients suffering from certain diseases.

Risk level	General population	Patients with specified diseases
1		tetanus
2		cancer, diabetes, peptic ulcer
3	cancer	arthritis
4	peptic ulcer	
5	arthritis, diabetes	whooping cough
6		
7	whooping cough, tetanus	
8		

DR MANN: This table (Table 19) was shown to a group of GPs. There was a fairly marked reaction, indicating that the patients are not interested at all, but are interested in culpability. They think that going to the doctor is something that should be associated with a benign outcome and are not interested in comparisons of absolute or relative risk. Table 19 shows a type of unicohort number, which has previously been made available. Most of the data are available in Hansard. These are four NSAIDs which have been the subject of action in the last 5 years, where the information is in the public domain about the marketing period so there is an actual time base. The number of deaths presumed to be drug-related is in the public literature. The unicohort number is the number of prescriptions for one death.

The worst case is Osmosin. The unicohort number is 10000 prescriptions, not patients, and presumably there are at least two confounding factors: on the one hand under-reporting and on the other hand many patients receive more than one prescription. We are, therefore, talking about a number of patients which is out of the reach of the controlled clinical study.

DR FITZGERALD: Could I re-open the question of experts not knowing

Table 19

NSAID	Market period (months)	Number of deaths	Prescriptions per 1 death
Opren	22	61	24 590
Zomax	23	7	128 571
Osmosin	10	40	10 000
Flosint	12	8	15 000

anything about risk. I feel slightly uncomfortable with the general view that it is the public that determines the level of risk.

PROFESSOR RAWLINS: It is not the level but the acceptance of risk that is determined by the public. There is a great difference between what the level of risk is and what the acceptance of that risk is.

DR FITZGERALD: Can we move out of the drug area. If an issue has been raised about the safety of a particular motorway bridge, I don't think I would ask anyone other than an engineer to give a view of the issue. I don't see that going to the public is going to help in any way with regard to the safety of the motorway.

PROFESSOR RAWLINS: The engineer will tell you it is 10^7 or 10^9, and it is up to you to decide whether it is safe enough to cross.

DR URQUHART: The insurance industry, historically, taught the doctors that benign essential hypertension wasn't benign. That result came from a large actuarial study of 350 000 people who had applied for life insurance, had their blood pressure measured, and 25 years later the data were put together. They were published in 1959 and re-done in 1979 with more recent data. There was also the interesting study published by the company State Mutual, who took the first Surgeon General's report in 1963 and built a marketing programme for discounting life insurance for non-smokers. They sold US$12 billion of insurance, US$5 billion to smokers and US$7 billion to non-smokers, and reported the result of 781 deaths in 1981. They found a 2.7 relative risk factor for coronary heart disease deaths and a 15-fold risk factor for lung cancer, and overall a 2.2-fold difference in mortality. This illustrates an enormous information gathering capability compared to the pharmaceutical industry. It was terrorized by the thalidomide disaster and began to diversify into other industries – Squibb bought a candy factory, Warner-Lambert bought a bakery and Eli Lilly bought Elizabeth Arden Cosmetics. No-one went into the information intensive industry which allies what the drug business has become. Perhaps there is a natural link between the 400-year-old information intensive insurance industry and the pharmaceutical industry which has not been explored, as illustrated by the fact that there is no-one here from the insurance industry.

CHAIRMAN: The facts on which the insurance industry is based are the facts the Colin Dollery's of this world have accumulated. All the insurance industry has done is to put some monetary value on it.

DR URQUHART: Sometimes it is the other way around, as with the hypertension story – the insurance people figured it out before the doctors did. The insurance industry is capable of aggregating much larger numbers of people than any of us could do. It does, however, have a number of flaws and does not solve all the problems.

PROFESSOR DOLLERY: In particular, it is very far from a random sample because insurance companies reject all the people with substantially increased risk.

DR CAVALLA: Could I attempt to correlate Professor Rawlins with Dr Urquhart because I think they are both right in their way but they see the problem from different sides. A very erudite individual in the risk–benefit field is Professor Cleggs who was at ICI, and particularly interested in toxic and explosive risk in the chemical industry. He pointed out, and no-one has refuted him, that the public is risk-illiterate, they simply cannot understand risk. Dr Urquhart was correct when he said that the public was at the stage of a 7-year-old child unable to identify the difference in weight between a pound of feathers and a pound of lead. I think the reason why Dr Urquhart brings in the insurance industry is because it is 'street wise' and it is their business to understand risk. On the other hand, the medical profession is, in my view, at times quite dismissive of risk. They will encourage their patients to adopt procedures, particularly in surgery, which are very risk intensive and the benefit is problematic. However, the medical profession are very concerned about risks of medicines because in a way they see them as coming between themselves and the patient.

DR SNELL: The factor that has not yet been discussed is time. Time is of the essence when it comes to making regulatory and manufacturing decisions about a drug. There is not time to collect the insurance statistics where the time-scale is over 25 years or a generation. The problem we are faced with is a very short time-scale in which to make a risk–benefit decision. The PMS studies described today are not quick enough to do this, nor are the large-scale clinical trials and outcome studies. We do need something else. Prescription Event Monitoring is getting nearer; Professor Inman's studies are capable of quite quick answers, but only in specified types of drugs.

PROFESSOR INMAN: Only when the drug has been on the market long enough to give us 10000 patients, which can be a long time.

DR SNELL: Yes. We do need something else, and I hope Stuart Walker is going to tell us at some point today what he is doing in the field of record linkage towards trying to find a more rapid answer to this problem.

PROFESSOR RAWLINS: Intuitively, formal cost–benefit analysis seems to be the most satisfactory way, but as Colin pointed out very clearly it is extraordinarily difficult because you have pears and apples. There have been two approaches to try and get around the problem. One is to put a monetary value on benefit and risk and there are economic ways of doing this. The other way, and I think it is the Economics unit at York who have done this, is to produce a sort of Richter scale on a logarithmic basis of benefits and risks from medicines. I wonder what Colin's views of this analytical way of trying to get around the problem are.

PROFESSOR DOLLERY: I have thought a lot about the monetary scale. Some of you may have read the enquiry carried out some years ago into the siting of the third London Airport, when Maplin Sands was in contention. They tried to put costs on, for example, the increased amount of time people would spend on travelling to the airport, i.e. several million people spending an hour or two a year in travelling. It turned out that these indirect costs came out as a very large fraction of the whole cost of building the airport. However, I felt sympathetic towards a critique of that report because although it is superficially attractive to ask people what money value they would put on not having a stroke over the next year, on not dying suddenly over the next year or not developing gout, thus reducing everything to a single scale, I am not sure whether it actually helps very much.

CHAIRMAN: What you are saying is that you are only looking at benefits to an individual group and omit to look at total benefits and total costs to the community as a whole.

PROFESSOR DOLLERY: I have calculated that the drug cost per stroke patient saved in the MRC trial where we used the cheapest form was only about £3000. That sounds a pretty good buy, but then as you say you have to start weighing all the other things.

PROFESSOR RAWLINS: They weren't fatal strokes, were they, so you have to add in the community care costs.

PROFESSOR GRAHAME-SMITH: Can I make a comment about Colin's exposition of the MRC trial. It seems to me that that has been an extremely useful trial because it could have shown that if you didn't treat mild hypertension you were almost, as a doctor, criminally negligent. That is not how it has turned out. The benefits are marginal and, before the trial was published, when faced with the individual patient with all the personal variables that patients have, you may have felt obliged to treat the patient's blood pressure. Now you don't end up feeling guilty for not treating hypertension and it seems to me that this is quite an important conclusion.

PROFESSOR DOLLERY: The point is that I want to prevent strokes and myocardial infarction and I am sad that we didn't do more in preventing myocardial infarction even if it cost something.

PROFESSOR VON WARTBURG: I would like to come back to the issue of real risks versus perceived risks. I have often been puzzled by the fact that people feel that society is based on a rational model and if one knew all the realities then social responses would be rational responses. So if we were to know all the risks and their relationship, severity, etc. then society by means of regulatory authorities would behave rationally. All the experience we have in other circles shows us that society is not necessarily based on this rational model of decision making in politics. To me the question boils down to 'Does society react to real risks or does it react to perceived risks? Does it react in a rational or an emotional way?'. In my experience, both as a teacher and as being from the pharmaceutical industry, usually the reaction results in a response to published opinion, not necessarily to public opinion. After a reaction has occurred, one goes back to the expert for an opinion. One of my first concerns would be to have more rationality put into published opinion because this has an impact on public opinion and on political action. If it is true that perceptions become reality, then at least within the pharmaceutical industry one also has to take note that such perceptions can be changed if one does it the right way. As far as risks are concerned, the perceptions are always being created in an individualized fashion, but in terms of benefits it is always a collective argument. The man in the street or journalist can deal very well with the individualized type of risk, but he cannot deal very well with the collective approach to benefit. I think, at least as far as the pharmaceutical industry is concerned, one should go more in the direction of also showing the individual benefits which have occurred and give some kind of counter-momentum to this rather emotional based perception of risk and the political reactions to it.

PROFESSOR TEELING-SMITH: I think Professor Dollery's account of the mild to moderate hypertension trial has focussed our attention on a very central issue to today's discussion. We are talking about the possibility of saving about 1000 strokes a year, and Colin has correctly told us that patients, not surprisingly, actually want that. Supposing aircraft crashes occurred 20 times a year and each one resulted in 50 people being seriously injured or crippled for the rest of their life, not killed. The aircraft industry would be in disarray. This situation is also being faced in the medical field, where it is being said that we won't treat because 1% of people may, for example, become impotent. David has actually said this gives the doctor justification for not treating. I disagree with this, but I think it does give the doctor a rational opportunity to discuss with the patient whether or not to treat. The doctor is faced with an ethical responsibility to put the question in simple terms to the patient.

DR IRVINE: Having taken part in the hypertension trial in my own practice, patients are now questioning me as to what the next stage is and what the results mean, particularly for themselves. It has been helpful to me as a clinician to have a better understanding than I had before the trial started of what the relative risks and benefits actually are and of the natural history of hypertension. This is the starting point of the decision which leads on to the next stage. It is a dialogue or negotiation between patient and doctor in which the values that Mike Rawlins was talking about really begin to come into play. It is a fact of life that people are far less concerned about dying, especially if it can be quick, than about the effects of morbidity. Stroke is a particular example, where the thought of lying disabled is far worse than the instant coronary. In my experience to date with the dozen or so people in this group, if there is a chance of reducing the effect of stroke without any serious consequences to their health they want it. That is how they judge and, given the balance as it looks to me, that is the sort of judgement that I as a doctor have gone along with.

CHAIRMAN: We have been particularly fortunate to have been allowed to study the natural history and response of mild hypertension so thoroughly. There are a number of instances where therapeutic intervention was initiated as a result of public demand rather than scientific knowledge. Cervical cytology is a good example where, because of cancerophobia, a decision was made to institute screening before knowing how worthwhile it really is.

DR CROMIE: Dr Irvine, how many of the patients that came back were you able to persuade to give up smoking? Surely the evidence shows that that is the number one priority irrespective of therapy.

DR IRVINE: That is a separate question. We have a clinical policy within the practice that anyone who comes in contact with any patients who smoke is advised to use any opportunity to persuade them not to. The key thing is to have the data in the patient record.

DAME ELIZABETH: Dr Irvine, do you ask your patients whether they drink? One has the impression that doctors are very coy about asking patients this. Yet in many ways alcohol is a greater killer.

DR IRVINE: You are absolutely right. We have only plucked up the courage in the last couple of years to declare the same kind of policy for alcohol as for cigarettes. It is actually surprising how forthcoming people are when it becomes part of routine questioning, unless they have something particular to conceal. Two basic pieces of data we want to know about our practice population are whether they smoke and whether they drink, because there are so many related conditions, causes of mortality and especially morbidity.

DR FITZGERALD: I wonder if Dr Mann would like to expand on the question of culpability, because this raised an unexpected flavour. Do patients, when they go to the doctor, believe that drugs are not a question of relative safety but of absolute safety and, therefore, the doctor is culpable if a mishap does occur? Clearly this is now becoming a major issue. The pharmaceutical industry as a whole is in serious problems about obtaining any insurance at the present time, particularly in North America. Is it possible to link these together, the idea of culpability and absolute safety for which the patient has an expectation whether generated by the media or the doctor?

DR MANN: My remark was born out of talking to a group of GPs about the problem. They may not be typical, but they are finding patients are worried about an emotive issue which they have described as culpability. The patient is not equating this phenomenon with a risk, for example, of being hit by lightning on a golf course, which is no-one's fault. The patient appears to be taking the view that he expects a benign outcome when he goes to the doctor and if he doesn't it worries him. This means we are involved with the highly emotive issue of culpability, an awkward but real part of the problem of drug risk. We are concerned with absolute and relative risk. I see us saddled with a problem of numbers of a kind of magnitude that can be reached no other way than they are at the moment, a very difficult methodology to get at the hard science and a public education problem in that they do not perceive the issue the way in which we perceive it.

PROFESSOR GEORGE: We did a systematic survey in Southampton recently, and the level of awareness of common unwanted effects was very low even among medicine takers.

PROFESSOR LEE: Firstly, the opposite of rationality is not emotionalism; they are two different qualities. When we say the public is irrational, what we mean is that they have a different set of reasons than us, and I think it is important to bear this in mind. Secondly, relating to culpability, did the doctor know there was a risk involved? If he knew, did he have the ability to have avoided or prevented it? Did he intend to impose the risk? Did he profit from that intention to impose the risk? Does he customarily do this kind of thing or was it merely an aberration? For example, it makes a great deal of difference, both in the perceived severity of the situation and the culpability that will be attached, whether a lump of wood that falls on your head broke off accidentally from a tree or whether someone cast it down. In relation to chemical hazards of the major catastrophe kind, the insurance market has reached its limit and is opting out. It will soon have to opt out of liability insurance for practitioners.

DR JONES: This is a very specialized audience and to some extent we are all obsessed with risk. I would like to ask the clinicians whether, when they are prescribing for patients, the patients actually ask if the drug will harm them and what the risks of taking it are. My own presumption is that patients are not as worried as we think they are.

CHAIRMAN: It depends very much on the type of disease being treated.

DR JONES: Particularly the general practitioners, who are doing most of the prescribing.

PROFESSOR DOLLERY: It depends also on the country. If you are doing a ward round in the United States you are much more likely to be cross-examined by the patient about the potential adverse effects of the drug than you are here. However, if you compare here now with here 15 years ago, particularly the middle class patient, then you are more likely to be asked such questions than before.

DR URQUHART: I think awareness is exemplified by the fact that there are 13 million copies of 'The Physician's Desk Reference' out in the United States market.

PROFESSOR VERE: I think patients' main worry in East London, expressed to us as physicians working there, seems to be dependence, even though most of the drugs involved have no connection with drug dependence induction whatsoever. It is purely because of what is in the media.

PROFESSOR GEORGE: 62% of Southampton residents feel that not enough is explained about medicines by doctors or pharmacists.

PROFESSOR GOLDBERG: I think Gerald has raised a very interesting question. In the past there has always been an expectation that a drug should be prescribed if a patient went to the doctor. Times have changed and in my own experience there is a greater acceptance, by the patient, if no drug is prescribed or if there are less drugs, because of this fear that has been raised by various experiences.

CHAIRMAN: I would like to thank this morning's speakers and all the discussants. I started by saying that the audience were as well informed as the speakers and I think it has become very evident from the splendid discussion we have had that has proven to be the case.

Session 3

Measuring the Benefits of Medicines

3.1 Clinical benefits

Dr J.D. Fitzgerald

Until about 40 years ago the methodology for measuring clinical benefits relied, to an unacceptable extent, upon conclusions based on clinical impression applied in a rather pragmatic fashion. Many forms of therapy were considered beneficial on the basis more of the status and authority of the proponent, rather than upon sound experimental principles. Physicians based their treatment choice upon what they had seen happen with the same intervention in one or two previous cases. The application of the elementary principles of experimental design, based upon valid statistical principles, has revolutionized the approach to the measurement of clinical benefit. The concept of having control and treated groups, which have the same characteristics in all relevant respects, eliminated observer bias and permitted valid generalizations about clinical interventions, based upon suitable samples of a particular disease. The activity of measuring the effects of therapeutic interventions in diseases to determine clinical benefit has expanded dramatically in the intervening years, and is one of the more important activities of clinical pharmacologists. A large body of data has accumulated in many disease areas supporting, or disproving, the possible clinical benefit of a large range of interventions, including not only drugs, but surgical, manipulative and other activities.

There is a general impression at this time that the science of measuring clinical benefit is in good shape, and anyone scanning the contents of this book would form the view that of all the topics for discussion, that of measuring clinical benefit is the least controversial, and that, in contemplating the risk/benefit equation, measuring benefit is the least of our problems. After all, governmental agencies have promulgated numerous texts or guidelines on measuring the benefit of drug intervention, and if consensus has been achieved in that setting, then the matter must surely be settled. In the next few pages I would like to raise some problems associated with such a widely held view.

An example of why I believe this topic is more debatable and uncertain than many believe is illustrated by some comments made at a recent clinical meeting. The case being presented was that of a 60-year-old man diagnosed as malignant hypertensive 7 years ago. In order to control his blood pressure, he was exposed to the inevitable range of antihypertensive drugs, and his very competent General Practitioner described the impact of each hospital recommendation for change in therapy upon the patient. There was impotence from diuretics or β-blockers; diabetes from diazoxide; hypoglycaemia due to tolbutamide; flushing and peripheral oedema from calcium antagonists, and so the list went on. During the 6 year illness he also had two strokes.

In the subsequent discussion, a consultant asked, 'With all you've been through, are you not sorry that you took the treatment in the first place?'. The patient looked in amazement at his General Practitioner, and mumbled something. His General Practitioner replied crisply, 'If you are asking would he rather be dead from his hypertension, the answer is no'.

Whilst you may regard this example as trivial, I suggest that it captures something of the dilemma of measuring clinical benefit, namely, what value system is to be applied in measuring benefit? I, therefore, propose to make some comments firstly upon benefit, its meaning and relevance, secondly, types of benefit, thirdly, the objectives in measuring clinical benefit, and finally, the need for a reappraisal of clinical benefit, which places a greater emphasis upon the patient's and society's values, rather than predominantly the clinician's.

In approaching this topic it is good practice to define the terms used. By 'benefit', I mean the probability that something good will happen. Arising from this definition are the issues of who defines what is meant by 'something good'. Does the clinician's view of benefit coincide with that of the patient's? Clearly, in many areas of disease there is no debate. However, there are many areas, particularly in primary health care, where it is by no means clear that when a patient comes to the doctor, that what one doctor defines as illness, would necessarily be agreed by another. Thus, the issue of assessing and agreeing the degree of illness prior to intervention for benefit must be a considerable problem.

For example, a doctor asked to visit an old man, living in a flat who is cold, hungry and lonely, is faced with a difficult problem as to whether this man is ill in the currently accepted terminology. There are many potential interventions the doctor could make that could result in something good happening, but will the doctor's objectives be the same as that of the patient, or of the patient's relatives? One could argue that this is a poorly chosen example, since there is no clearly defined clinical condition. It is, however, a widespread human condition which requires improvement to bring about benefit.

Such considerations lead to the need to examine different types of possible benefit, and for ease of discussion I have suggested three categories. Firstly, palliative, in which the relief of symptoms is brought about without affecting the course of the disease, as for example, the use of analgesics in pain associated with malignant disease. Secondly, delay of disease progression as in the previously quoted example of malignant hypertension. Thirdly, the cure of disease, as in tuberculous meningitis, or *Escherichia coli* peritonitis.

If we take the first type of benefit, namely that of disease palliation, what are the issues in regard to measuring clinical benefit? For example, how is clinical benefit assessed, and who defines the criteria? How can individual needs be incorporated into a generalized view? What should be measured, and how should it be measured?

Some of the objectives in palliation are freedom from external interference, preservation of stamina and intellectual acuity, enjoyment of vocational and social activities. However, do the current assessment procedures incorporate these objectives? The management of symptomatic coronary artery disease illustrates some of these difficulties. For the past 10 years, there has been a prolonged debate concerning the relative merits of medical versus surgical therapy in angina pectoris. Because the elementary principles of experimental design and statistical principles were ignored in the early phases of coronary artery surgery, there were deep divisions as to its value. The coronary artery surgery study (CASS) reported in 1983 that in comparison with medical therapy there was an overall benefit[1].

An overall analysis showed (Figure 17) that when comparing medical versus surgical therapy, surgery was better in the sense that there was less pain, better exercise tests, and less drug therapy. However, there was no

SURGERY	NO DIFFERENCE
Less pain	Survival
Better exercise tests	Activity limitation
Less drug therapy	Employment status
	Recreational status

CLASSICAL PARAMETERS ALL SHOW BENEFIT
YET INTERPRETATION IS CONTROVERSIAL

Figure 17 Coronary Artery Surgery Study – medical v. surgical therapy

difference in overall survival at 5 years, in activity limitation, in employment status or in recreational status.

Thus, the classicial parameters used to assess clinical benefit all showed benefit, yet the interpretation of these results remains controversial. I would suggest that the dilemma facing us all is coming to an agreement on what constitutes clinical benefit.

When measuring clinical benefit, whatever method is used, judgement must be made by the investigator about its relevance to the purpose in hand. Amongst the principles underlying the methodology is, first of all, the assessment must be relevant to the patient need. In the case of anginal studies, by far the greatest weight is placed by investigators on the type of observation just described, but are these observations strictly relevant to patient need? Whatever measurement is made, standardization of scales is essential and the basis of the scaling must be specified. Of equal importance is that subjective assessments need not correlate necessarily with biochemical and physical measurement. However, clearly their inter-relationship can be studied, but it is not essential to anchor subjective assessments to a perceived higher quality or 'more objective parameter' of biochemical and physical measurements. In the case of the CASS study, there is no doubt that surgery does provide more impressive and established benefit in terms of reduction of incidence of pain. Also I am sure that in correctly selected patients there is little doubt that it is of important clinical benefit. However, when coming to pool the results of large studies in such diseases the problems of applying these results to the general anginal population are not eased if only treadmill, ECG and diary cards are used as recommended by the current E.E.C. guidelines.

If we turn now to the second category of potential benefit, namely delay of disease progression, there are two sub-categories here. Firstly, delay of progress in asymptomatic conditions, and secondly delay of progress in symptomatic conditions.

In the asymptomatic category, as exemplified by therapeutic inter-ventions for the management of severe hypertension, or severe hyper-lipidaemia, there has been intense debate over the past 10 years as to what constitutes clinical benefit. In the spectrum of hypertensive disease, it is universally accepted that reducing blood pressure in patients with malignant hypertension prolongs survival. This is one of the major achievements in the medical management of hypertension in the last 30 years, though its importance is not generally recognized outside the medical profession.

The reduction of diastolic blood pressure of more than 110 mmHg in patients will reduce the incidence of cerebral vascular accidents, but clearly does not eliminate them, only postpones them. Furthermore, it seems that there is no major impact on the main cause of death and disability in hypertension, namely myocardial infarction and sudden death. Even more contentious, of course, are the likely benefits to an individual patient of normalizing the serum cholesterol level from say 300 to 210 mg/100 ml. In both these conditions the epidemiological evidence is very persuasive, i.e. for an individual patient therapy is clearly indicated. These views are, however, based on the clinician's knowledge and perspective of the natural history of the disease. It is legitimate to ask whether these criteria are valid when it comes to the individual patient's point of view. As far as the individual patient is concerned, the criteria of clinical benefit for the management of asymptomatic diseases with serious prognosis remains a contentious issue and should be related to the patient's value system rather than the physician's.

If we turn now to the delay of disease progression in symptomatic conditions, for example rheumatoid arthritis or duodenal ulcer, here one might ask are the current criteria of benefit valid? In the case of duodenal ulcer for example, a pivotal observation required by regulatory authorities is the rate of ulcer healing following the therapeutic intervention. However, there is no clear correlation between symptomatic relief and rate of ulcer healing, and neither is there a relationship between ulcer relapse rate and rate of ulcer healing.

It might be interesting to debate the proposition that if the intervention had no effect on the rate of ulcer healing in comparison with placebo, but gave instant relief of all symptoms, was this a clinically beneficial intervention on the assumption that there were no other unwanted side-effects? Similarly, in the case of rheumatoid arthritis, there are numerous indices of the arrest of disease progression, based primarily on serial radiological assessment. I would suggest, however, that there are many unanswered questions in this difficult area, and whilst the regulatory guidelines for the evaluation of drugs in rheumatoid arthritis represent the best current advice on the state of the art of assessment, they remain imperfect. Similar comments could apply to a whole range of disease categories in which the intervention may delay disease progression. It seems reasonable to ask, therefore, has the search for objective data and its statistical manipulation distorted the relevance of the selected measurement?

The final category is that of the cure or prevention of disease. In general, in this area one is on firmer ground. For example, if one examines the influence of antibiotics in the management of TB meningitis or coliform peritonitis, there is clear-cut proof of benefit from any point of view.

Similarly, in the area of prevention, for example smallpox vaccination, a similar view would be held, and it is a sad criticism of our Western media that I have yet to see the banner headline indicating that smallpox has been eliminated as a clinical problem. Less clear-cut to some is, of course, the benefit of whooping cough vaccination. There is no doubt that it is a most valuable intervention, and the media-induced loss of confidence in this has subsequently been shown to have caused a marked increase in morbidity and mortality associated with pertussis infection[2]. The clear-cut proof of benefit from any point of view is not shared by the media and that can only be a matter of sadness.

In conclusion, I have attempted to raise a number of issues in the area of measuring clinical benefit. Possible topics for debate are, firstly the approach using categorization of clinical benefit, is it necessary or helpful in the discussion? Of greater importance to the debate is, who is the arbiter of clinical benefit – the doctor, the patient or the regulatory agency? I would conclude with the motion that the measurement of clinical benefit is as complex and imperfect as that of risk assessment, though most people, if asked the question without discussion, would disagree with that statement.

References

1. CAGS Principal Investigators and their Associates (1983). Coronary artery surgery study (CAGG): a randomized trial of coronary bypass surgery. Survival data. *Circulation*, **68**, 934–50
2. Williams, W.O. (1985). Long-term sequelae of whooping cough. *Proc R. Soc. Med.*, **78**, 707–9

3.2 Economic benefits

Professor G. Teeling Smith

The economic benefits derived from the pharmaceutical industry take two broad forms. First, the use of medicines saves other types of health service costs, and these savings can be quantified in a number of ways. Second, the existence and activities of the industry make a direct economic contribution to the wealth of the country, in just the same way as other industries manufacturing any other types of goods for home consumption and for export. This paper deals with these two types of economic contribution, and concludes that in 1982 the pharmaceutical industry in England and Wales made a net contribution to government finance of at least £1100 million.

Based on this calculation, it is argued that the government's measures to restrict the activities and the sales of the pharmaceutical industry in Britain could result in an overall cost to the government exchequer, instead of saving the government money. Thus the government's insistence on viewing pharmaceutical expenditures in isolation as a 'problem' of public expenditure is economically unsound.

Looking first at the direct savings achieved by the use of pharmaceuticals, in the 1950s and 1960s it was usual to estimate the overall economic savings in three ways[1]. The first was to calculate the savings in hospital costs as a result of reductions in the numbers of occupied bed-days. The second was to calculate the reduction in numbers of working days lost due to certified sickness absence, and to estimate the economic benefits in terms of increased production and reduced sickness benefit payments. The third type of saving resulted from reduced mortality. For example in the case of tuberculosis it could be estimated that the addition to the working population as a result of reduced tuberculosis mortality contributed £40 million to national wealth in 1962[2].

However in the 1980s the second and third of these types of saving – reduced 'sickness' absence and reduced mortality – are something of an illusion, and it is no longer appropriate to put so much emphasis on them in justifying the cost of pharmaceuticals in economic terms.

Taking sickness absences first, there are two reasons why it is now less relevant to include them in a 'cost–benefit' equation for the use of pharmaceuticals. First, although individual medicines can still show remarkable reductions in work lost through sickness, in general in all western countries the overall statistics for absences attributed to sickness are showing an increase. This is because people are now more readily able to afford to take time off work for more trivial sickness. They often receive their full pay during an absence attributed to sickness, and in many other cases they will receive fairly generous payments from their social security scheme to compensate for lost earnings. Certainly the causes recorded for sickness absence suggest that it is the more trivial 'diagnoses' which are responsible for the increase. Serious illness often shows a reduction in the numbers of days of work lost – and this is usually due to more effective medication[3]. The willingness of people to take time off work for more trivial symptoms does, in a very real sense, indicate an improvement in the quality of life. People no longer need to struggle into work when they feel 'one degree under'. However, this improvement is hard to measure in economic terms, and hence for this reason no attempt has been made here to quantify the effects of medicines on either productivity or overall wellbeing.

Second, in relation to sickness absence, there is now the problem that unemployment and sickness absence interact in their economic effect. Often if a person is made well enough to work through effective therapy he or she may do no more than add to the pool of unemployed persons. Hence, for this reason also, the 'savings' from any reductions in sickness absence would have to be treated with caution.

Turning to reductions in mortality, similar considerations apply. In the 1950s dramatic advances in the treatment of tuberculosis and other infections saved many young lives, and added to the effective pool of available labour, practically all of which could be fully employed. However, in the 1980s the situation is different. First, even when a young death is prevented by effective medication the person whose life is saved may do more than add to the numbers out of work.

But more fundamentally, most medicines in the 1980s have their greatest effects in improving the quality of life – in reducing painful symptoms and disability – rather than in preventing premature mortality. Most deaths now occur after the age of retirement. Once again, it may eventually be possible to quantify the benefits of pharmaceuticals in terms of quality of life in precise economic terms. But in the meantime it is prudent to exclude the effects of changing patterns of mortality from an economic analysis of the benefits from the use of modern medicines.

On the other hand, no such problems arise with savings due to the reduction in hospital treatments as a result of the effective use of pharmaceuticals. Between 1957 and 1982, the total number of occupied hospital beds in England and Wales fell from 420000 to 295000. This reduction in beds in 1982 can be estimated – as a 'ball-park' figure – to be responsible for savings of £3 billion.

Although most of this reduction could probably fairly be attributed to the use of modern medicines, it is possible to make more conservative and more precise estimates of their economic effect on the hospital service. Table 20 shows six diseases where the development of effective medicines has led specifically to a reduction in the need for hospital treatment. Overall, total hospital bed days for these six conditions fell by 50% between 1957 and 1982. This reduction has been achieved in a variety of ways. Thus in asthma, for example, an increase in the number of patients receiving hospital care has been more than offset by a fall of more than two thirds in the duration of hospital stay. The drop in bed days for bronchitis, on the other hand, is a function of both fewer in-patient admissions and a halving of the stay in hospital. Table 21 shows the

Table 20 Total hospital bed days for six diseases in 1957 and 1982 .

Disease	1957	1982
Asthma	394331	297381
Epilepsy	500053	247352
Glaucoma	148969	89096
Hyptertensive disease	1204277	185510
Bronchitis	1262028	471459
Skin diseases	1122385	996204
Total	4632043	2287002

Note: In 1982 the data source from which bed days are calculated, the Hospital In-patient Enquiry, referred to England only

Source: Hospital In-patient Enquiry for 1957 and 1982

Table 21 Financial savings from the reduction in hospital bed days 1957–1982

	Bed days 1957	Bed days 1982	Savings in bed days 1957–1982	Savings in* hosp. costs (£ Million)
Six diseases	4632043	2287002	2345041	176
Respiratory TB	6886552	106323	6780229	509
Infectious diseases excluding Resp. TB	2766190	553947	2232243	167
Mental illness	52487000***	25162370	27324630	847
				1699

*   Average daily cost in acute hospitals with 51 beds or more in 1982/83: £75
   Average daily cost in mental illness hospitals in 1982: £31
** 1959 data

Source: Hospital In-patient Enquiry for 1957 and 1982

estimated savings in 1982 hospital costs resulting from the reductions in hospital bed days for these six diseases and for respiratory tuberculosis, other infectious disease and mental illness. Both respiratory tuberculosis and mental illness are classic examples of pharmaceutical progress dramatically reducing the need for hospital treatment. Tuberculosis was very nearly eliminated, and Figure 18 shows how a previously rising trend in the number of occupied mental illness beds was reversed by the introduction of chlorpromazine in 1954. It was only some years later that changes in the law recognized the new scope for treatment of mentally ill patients on a voluntary and increasingly community-orientated basis.

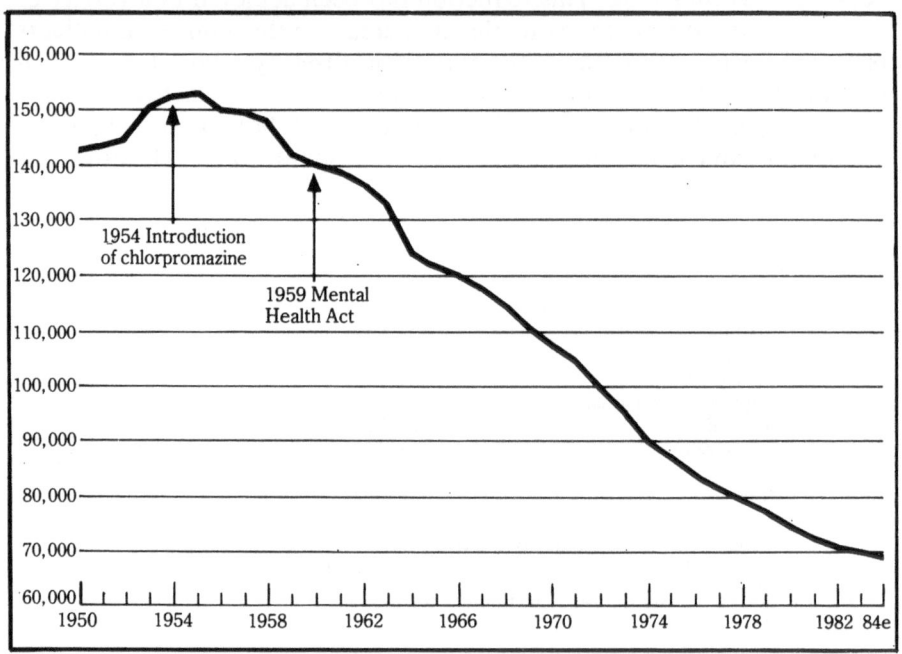

Figure 18 Number of in-patients in mental hositals. England 1950-1984. Sources: DHSS Annual Reports and DHSS Illness and Handicap Hospitals Statistics

Taking these nine diseases alone, the reduction in occupied beds between the second half of the 1950s and 1982 represents a saving of £1699 million for the NHS in England and Wales.

It has been argued in the past, when similar calculations have been presented, that they ignore the other side of the coin – the hospital costs of treating adverse reactions to medicines. In order to take account of this criticism, these costs have also been estimated for this paper.

Table 22 shows the proportion of hospital discharges and deaths and of hospital bed days attributable to 'poisoning and toxic effects of medicinal

Table 22 Discharges from or deaths in hospital attributable to poisoning and toxic effects of medicinal agents

Year	As per cent of all discharges and deaths	As per cent of all bed days
1977	2.43	0.45
1978	2.24	0.44
1979	2.04	0.40
1980	1.95	0.35
1981	1.92	0.37
1982	1.87	0.36
1983	1.63	0.30

Source: Hospital In-patient Enquiry, various years

agents' between 1971 and 1983. It is immediately apparent from these figures that a steady decline has been taking place over this period. As a result, hospital discharges and deaths due to this specific cause had fallen to 85 660 in 1982 (the year common to the other analyses contained in this paper) and hospital bed days summed to 197 000. It may, therefore, be calculated that hospitalization caused by poisoning and toxic effects of medicinal agents cost £15 million in 1982.

It should be pointed out, however, that the figures for discharges and deaths include an unknown but probably substantial number of cases of deliberate self-poisoning[4]. Unintentional adverse effects of medicines may, therefore, account for only a relatively small proportion of the cases included in the category 'poisoning and toxic effects of medicinal agents'. Yet it is also true that patients admitted to hospital for other specific causes may, during their stay, experience an adverse effect from a medicine prescribed to treat their original illness. It is not possible to estimate from the available data the numbers involved in such episodes nor the extent of additional hospital stay thereby required. However, a recent paper from Switzerland suggests that 1% of hospital cases may be due to the serious adverse effects of medicine[5]. If this proportion is applied to the total number of hospital bed days calculated from the Hospital In-patient Enquiry it may be estimated that serious adverse reactions to medicines cost the hospital sector £41 million in 1982. This figure is almost three times the estimate presented earlier but, as will be shown below, it still has little impact on the very favourable cost–benefit ratio for pharmaceuticals.

Just as it is possible to estimate the economic benefits of pharmaceuticals from several different standpoints, the costs can also be calculated in various ways. In 1982, the total cost of the family practitioner pharmaceutical services including dispensing fees was £1361 million for England and Wales. Including the costs of all hospital medicines increases this total to £1602 million. However, out of this latter total, pharmaceutical manufacturers received only £1225 million. This is the figure which it seems most appropriate to use in producing a cost–benefit equation for the pharmaceutical industry's contribution to the National Health Service. On this basis, and employing the greater of the two hospitalized adverse reaction costs (£41 million), the pharmaceutical industry's products yielded net savings to the NHS of £433 million in 1982.

However, the simple cost–benefit equation, showing the government's saving in respect of the NHS hospital service from the use of pharmaceuticals, does not complete the picture. The pharmaceutical industry and its employees also pay taxes.

In addition to the pharmaceutical industry's sales to the National Health Service in 1982, it had export sales of £1008 million. In a recent publication from the Office of Health Economics, an attempt was made to estimate the taxes paid by the pharmaceutical industry on the profits made from its home and export sales, and also the taxes paid on earnings by its employees[6]. Together, these figures represent the direct income received by the Inland Revenue from the pharmaceutical industry's operations in the United Kingdom. The estimate was made by using the assumption that the pharmaceutical industry and its employees would pay the same average taxes as applied to British industry as a whole. Although this method of estimation cannot give a definitive figure, it is unlikely to vary greatly from the actual taxes paid.

For 1982, for the United Kingdom as a whole, it was estimated that the pharmaceutical industry contributed £760 million in taxes. As the major estimates in this paper relate to England and Wales only, it is appropriate to reduce this UK figure *pro rata* on a population basis to £665 million.

Thus taking the total picture of the government's expenditure and income and savings from the operation of the pharmaceutical industry in England and Wales, it can be conservatively estimated that the industry made a net contribution to the exchequer of £1098 million in 1982.

It can, of course, be argued that some of the benefits which have been discussed, such as the conquest of tuberculosis, are historical; whereas the continued expenditure on pharmaceuticals is a current expense. To some extent this is the case, but it remains true that the savings from past therapeutic triumphs are still just as real today as they were 20 years ago. Nevertheless, the Office of Health Economics is now concentrating more on measurements of the improvement in quality of life, so that hard economic benefits in those terms can be set against the expenditure of recently introduced medicines whose greatest contribution is to reduce suffering and disability. These 'quality of life' studies are discussed in other papers at this meeting, and, therefore, lie outside the scope of the present discussion. However, even taking the strictly financial economic picture above, there are causes for concern in recent political developments. Since 1983 successive moves by the government in relation to the pharmaceutical industry have been solely concerned to reduce the size of the National Health Service payments to the pharmaceutical industry, by reducing its profitability, by limiting its sales through the National Health Service, and by attempting to influence the industry's expenditure on such items as research, administration and sales promotion.

Whereas the government's attempts to restrict public expenditure – and hence taxation – are wholly commendable, it would appear that in relation to the pharmaceutical industry they could have been dangerously shortsighted. The pharmaceutical industry is precisely the sort of high technology, high-added value industry which the British economy needs. This paper has indicated that Britain is not only benefiting in general from the presence of its pharmaceutical industry, but also that Britain's exchequer is making a very substantial positive gain from the industry's activities and achievements.

Measures to restrict the pharmaceutical industry's activities in Britain cannot, therefore, be seen only in terms of a potential reduction in NHS pharmaceutical expenditure. They must be judged in the light of the industry's overall economic contribution. A smaller, less profitable and less effective pharmaceutical industry in Britain could actually *increase* costs to the government, rather than reducing them. A 'cheap-drug' policy, such as the government seems to have tried to introduce since 1983, could be very expensive in the medium to long term not only in human terms for NHS patients, but also in economic terms for British taxpayers.

References

1. Teeling Smith, G. (1963). *The Human and Economic Contribution of Drugs.* (London) Association of the British Pharmaceutical Industry)
2. Office of Health Economics, (1962). *Progress Against Tuberculosis,* (London: OHE)
3. Wells, N.E.J. (1981). *Sickness Absence; A Review* (London: OHE)
4. Wells, N.E.J. (1981). *Suicide and Deliberate Self-Harm* (London: OHE)
5. Pedrone, G. (1984). Drugs and Adverse Reactions: In Lindgren, B. (ed.) *Pharmaceutical Economics,* (Lund: Swedish Institute for Health Economics)
6. Chew, R, Teeling-Smith, G. and Wells, N.E.J. (1985). *Pharmaceuticals in Seven Nations,* (London: OHE)

3.3 Psycho-social benefits

Dr C. R. B. Joyce

INTRODUCTION

This paper is about the problems of collecting and using information on the psycho-social benefits from all drugs, not just those used in psychiatry.

The reason for collecting the information must be carefully defined at the start. Is it intended for the regulatory authority? Is it to help the choice of treatment for the individual patient? Or to provide a basis for management decisions by the company producing the medicine? The kind of information collected, and the weight to be put upon it, will differ depending upon the purpose, and so will the methods. Nord-Larsen distinguishes three general classes of method for estimating economic costs and benefits: those based on diagnoses or symptoms, on 'global subjective values of health status'; and on functional status or disability[1]. A similar categorization of methods can be fitted to studies of psycho-social benefits. Janke, writing about cancer studies, notes that very different methodologies are needed for making predictions about subjects (patient management) on one hand and about drugs (explanatory studies) on the other [2]. The way in which information is combined, and decisions eventually arrived at, is at the present time the most unsatisfactory aspect of the process. Most people are better at collecting information than at knowing what to do with it when they have it.

Psychological benefits are those that arise from and affect the individual's own functioning – sensing, perceiving, thinking, feeling and acting, especially insofar as these have the self itself as object. Social benefits are those that accrue to:

(1) The individual functioning as a member of a group, of whatever size;
(2) The group itself, or
(3) Society as a whole (an unsatisfactory concept).

99

As Dr Fitzgerald and Professor Teeling Smith have already covered each end of this very broad spectrum, one may well ask if anything is left to discuss? Certainly, not the traditional aspects of tolerability and efficacy, important as these undoubtedly are. They have largely, though not exclusively, to do with the understanding of the disease process, its control and modification, whereas psycho–social benefit is concerned with the understanding of the patient – the patient's self-perception and self-understanding – which is now usually referred to as quality of life.

QUALITY OF LIFE RESEARCH

Figure 19 gives an idea of the explosive increase in interest in 'quality of life' from the medical literature. Alexander and Willems (1981) believe that, until the 1960s, the term really meant 'quantity of life', so materialistic were the aspects chiefly considered[3]. In the 20 years since 1966, however, when the phrase seems first to have been used in something like its present sense, or senses, the annual number of papers indexed by the United States National Library of Medicine that mentioned 'quality of life' in title or keywords has increased from one to more than 350, giving a total of some 2000 or more at present. A majority of these consider the still fairly rudimentary theory of the subject, or give 'how to' guidelines, rather than reporting results. This paper will, alas, be yet another; our own group is now running its first experimental studies.

At least four main attitudes to the quality of life can be made out. The pessimistic view is that any change affecting life quality is always for the worse. The sceptical is that the concept is used so broadly and imprecisely that it has no meaning, and can even be regarded as a gimmick. The conservative view is that there is nothing new in it, because the doctor's task has always been to improve the quality of life of the patient. A fourth point of view, however, is that quality of life describes a new way of evaluating medical intervention. It uses new kinds of measurement to capture new information that is important for the patient, for the practice of medicine and for the place of health care in society. This attitude is positive, constructive and productive. Culyer believes that there are already 'scholarly techniques of sufficient sophistication' for establishing valid health indicators that can be 'far more widely incorporated into ... medical and epidemiological work, especially clinical trials' than has so far been done[4]. Interestingly, Mattson and her colleagues of the AMIS and B-HAT groups have shown that participation in these trials, as such, may have produced greater benefit than the degree of physical improvement experienced from the nominal treatment[5].

There is a need to define quality of life. Here I shall be pragmatic, or, perhaps, cowardly. Optimal life quality might be equated with the WHO

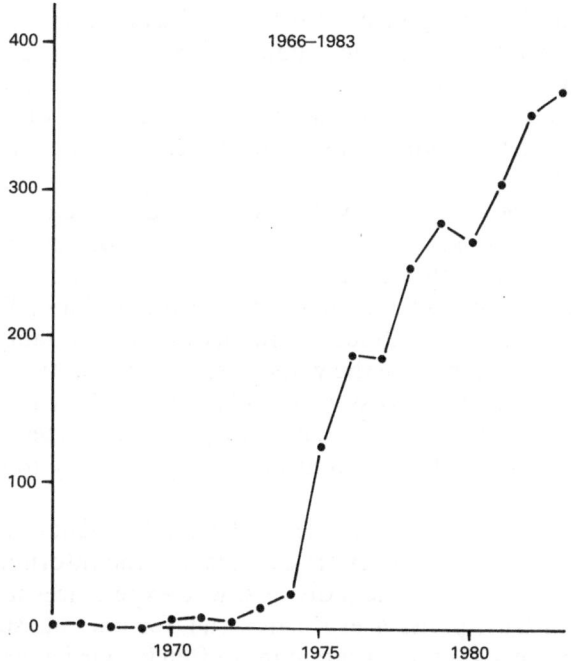

Figure 19   Publications regarding quality of life retrievable from *Medline*

definition of perfect health as a state of complete bodily, mental and social well-being, were such a definition not so idealistic as to be unattainable. It seems more useful to define life quality (similarly to the way in which some still define intelligence) as that which is measured by measurements of quality of life. As with intelligence, it is essential to say exactly what those tests are, what they are intended to measure and in what sense the results matter.

MEASURING PSYCHO-SOCIAL BENEFITS

The individual as the unit of study

The spectrum of possible enquiries and methods runs from experimental investigation of the individual to sociological surveys of what the relevant groups within a society do, or think should be done, in regard to life quality. At one end, there have been attempts to measure the 'happiness' of the individual[6], moving through more precise definitions of well-being, beliefs about health, economic studies of cost–risk trade-offs, to the formulation of statements about health policy at the other. The latter are concerned, whether explicitly or not, with the allocation of resources that are inevitably limited; individuals, as taxpayers, patients and voters, are again involved.

Information about the individual can be described at successively higher levels, from observations on elemental behaviours and symptoms through more elaborate, grouped measures of change, arriving at physical, psychological, social and economic 'dimensions'. The final level may be a single statement, about the quality of life, or quality of survival. (One might think death to be the worst case – zero quality, in the absence of life – were it not that Rosser and Watts have shown that there are indeed states worse than death[7].) Laboratory and clinical tests form part of the explanatory network, but contribute only indirectly to the measurement of life quality.

Specialists are involved at all times in the development of methods; but, in the end, only the patient report can provide the information needed. Each life is different. Only the individual who experiences it can judge its quality. This is true, perhaps especially true, for patients suffering from severe psychiatric disorders, where it may often be particularly difficult to get the patient's own evaluation, or where the consequences of doing so may be surprising. Physicians, family members or other individuals, whom American medical sociologists refer to as significant, may for various reasons be incapable of accurately reporting it, or may even ignore it altogether. Even the technique of 'social validation'[8], the combination of behavioural observation with verbal reports from 'significant others', may not be enough.

But although it is not sufficient for the physician alone to make the assessment, things may be worse if the patient does so, as some would apparently prefer[9,10]. Hartman points out that the major, perhaps the only, virtue of trying to obtain informed consent is that it ensures that the doctor talks to the patient[11] and – dare one hope? – even listens. Brinkley notes a related advantage in quality of life measurements: their use 'will constantly remind all concerned that it is the quality of the patient's life which is important – whether or not it can be measured accurately'[12]. There are methods that can provide consistent and explicit help in deciding how and even by whom such assessments are to be made[13].

Changes in the burden on the patient's family, etc are an important part of the social costs and benefits. Platt has given a very useful review of this area, including six scales designed for the purpose[14]. These, like scales devised for other purposes, lead to the discussion of fundamental matters.

Some basic methodological problems

Most researchers prefer observations to be as 'hard' as possible, but, as Fries has pointed out[15], in rheumatology at least some so-called 'soft' outcome measures now have demonstrably greater validity than other kinds of data long believed to be 'hard'. The distinction between hard and soft is not really useful; nor is the commonly used equivalent of subjective and objective. Instead, it appears better to separate external (or exteriorizable) from internal (or non-exteriorizable) information. If observations cannot be brought to the outside but remain private to the individual, they cannot be used for research. Emotions, attitudes, wishes, performances are all exteriorizable and provide acceptable scientific data.

But if the unit of study is always the individual, the unit of report, on the other hand, may sometimes be the individual and sometimes the group. How is the information to be combined and presented? Individual results may be expressed as 'indicators'[16], or as 'profiles'[17]. A crude illustration of the difference is that individual item scores on a rating scale of any kind constitute a profile, whereas the total score is an indicator of the overall strength of the variable studied. Culyer points out that the choice between indicators and profiles is still a major point of controversy amongst 'quality of life' workers[4]. This may in some part be because many of those who work with rating-scales are unfamiliar with more sophisticated methods[18,19]. These depend upon identifying items of information important to the individual, and in assessing how important these items are to him or her[20].

It is sometimes questioned if sophisticated measures of quality derived from an individual can be applied to a population sample, or even to other individuals. Rosser and her group[21,22], however, have provided evidence that, in certain circumstances, generalization of this kind is possible.

The observations must also be integrated with respect to time. Should one take 'snap-shots' at specific intervals, or sum the area under the 'quality of life' curve as is done with other time-sensitive measures? For example, Van Raaij, an economic psychologist, has found that people's intentions are better predictors of behaviour than their attitudes in snap-shot or cross-sectional studies, but attitudes predict better in time-series observations[23].

Preferences may change with time. This undoubtedly complicates the interactions and integration, but it must not be ignored[24]. There are of course many other problems. If a change of state is to be measured, there must be some basis of comparison. What should this be? The status of the individual 'now' versus the status 'then'; or the norms for his or her age, sex, etc; or an expression of personal standards; or a baseline representing an ideal state? Can the methods used be general or must they be modified to meet the specific character of the indication under study? What are the dimensions that must be included? How does one choose or invent a suitable method?

ASSESSING METHODS OF ASSESSMENT

Many scales have been developed and published. There are many good compilations and critical reviews[25], as well as the splendid quarterly annotated bibliography of unpublished as well as published work edited by Erickson[26]. Before re-inventing the wheel, it is worth while to see if someone else has invented any other means of transport for the road to be travelled[27].

The four sub-headings of this final section inevitably overlap. They are feasibility, relevance, validity and, for lack of a better work, connectedness.

Feasibility

It is obvious that if a study is not feasible, if it really cannot be carried out, it is a waste of time to try to do so; but it may be less obvious that executing a study only because it is feasible can be just as much a waste of time. If the method requires trained interviewers, it must be possible to have interviewers trained. Even the simplest method needs time, and many are not simple; the required time must be available. Some redundancy in the questions is usually helpful, but there must not be so much that the respondents are antagonized either on a single occasion or by multiple testing. Can the subjects understand the questions? Even if they do, are they able, for physical or other reasons, to answer them?

Relevance

Because drug effects on the quality of life may be positive as well as negative, tests, to be relevant, should be two-tailed; capable of revealing benefits as well as costs. Striking illustrations of this need have been given by Sugarbaker et al.[28], who observed more favourable responses to amputation than to chemotherapy for sarcoma of the tibia. Also by de Haes and van Krippenberg, who found that cancer patients do not necessarily judge their quality of life to be worse than that of the unaffected population[29].

The method of assessment must not only be appropriate to the indication and subjects, but also to their age, sex and culture (which often receives little more than lip service). It may need updating (questions about the quality of sexual life in two reports published as recently as 1978 were confined to *heterosexual* satisfaction). It must contain the dimensions agreed, by researcher and subject, to cover the kinds of knowledge sought – distress and disability may be enough[7], or six 'domains' of experience and seven of daily life, as in the Nottingham Health Profile[30], or even 40 may be required[22]. As Rosser says, comprehensiveness is elusive[31].

Validity

What does it need, or what does it mean to claim validity for a quality of life study? To make a real contribution to knowledge, it must have something more than 'face validity', i.e. superficial persuasiveness. The method of measurement really matters; Read and colleagues[32] compared three methods for assessing bypass patient outcome preferences, and found that the methods were 'not interchangeable'. That the concepts must be appropriate is obvious. Structural validity should be apparent from internal consistency; as revealed, for example, by factor analysis. But one vital aspect of validity is often ignored: the distinction between convergent and divergent validities (the demonstration that what is being studied is respectively the same as, or different from, something else). If quality of life is only another name for tolerability and/or efficacy, if its instruments only estimate something already being adequately measured, it is unnecessary. They should also demonstrate discriminant validity, the ability to show differences between treatments, patient groups, etc. Claims made for validation should be checked; sometimes they are no more than claims, and inadequately documented at that. The methods of analysis must be adequately described; and the use of the instrument by others than its authors should employ the recommended method of analysis, or reasons should be given for not having done so. Failures of such kinds may have occurred because this is an area for which even some of those who enter it have less than perfect respect.

Connectedness

Finally, by connectedness is meant the place of the method in the continuum of information, from complementing the results of clinical investigation at one end of the scale, to contributing meaningfully to the economic assessment of costs and benefits, and so to helping the formation of health policy, at the other. Reviewing 11 papers in medical sociology recommended by a peer group as being representative in terms of their 'intellectual content, insights into political philosophy, explana-

tory power, predictive power and opportunities for social improvements',
Culyer concluded that:

> the medical sociology literature is quite weak when judged by these
> criteria ... sociologists often seem to confuse issues that involve value
> judgements with ones that do not, and generally seem to display a
> disconcerting obsession with methodological issues of the most
> fundamental kind that has inhibited medical sociology from
> developing interesting analyses of many issues on which, in principle,
> it ought to have much to offer[33].

This paper may have manifested just such an obsession, although a
sociopharmacologist should have been as aware of this danger as of the
need to collect the information upon which the 'interesting analyses' are to
be based.

References

1. Nord-Larsen, M. (1983). What kind of health measure for what kind of purpose? In Culyer, A.J. (ed.). *Health Indicators*, pp. 101-9. (Oxford: Martin Robertson)
2. Janke, W. (1985). Clinical efficacy of drugs predicted from drug effects after short-term administration in animals, normal subjects and patients. *Neuropsychobiology*, 13, 53-4
3. Alexander, J.L. and Willems, E.P. (1981). Quality of Life: some measurement requirements. *Arch. Physic. Med. Rehabil.*, 62, 261-265
4. Culyer, A.J. (1983). Conclusions and recommendations. In Culyer, A.J. (ed.). *Health Indicators*, pp. 186-193. (Oxford: Martin Robertson)
5. Mattson, M.E., Curb, J.D., McArdle, R. and the AMIS and BHAT Research Groups (1985). Participation in a clinical trial: the patient's point of view. *Contr. Clin. Trials*, 6, 156-67
6. George, L.K. (1979). The Happiness Syndrome: methodological and substantive issues in the study of social-psychological well-being in adulthood. *Gerontologist*, 19, 210-16
7. Rosser, R.M. and Watts, V. (1975). A clinical classification of disability and distress and its application to the awards made by the courts in personal injury cases. *New Law J.*, 125, 323
8. Agran, M. and Martin, E.E. (1985). Establishing socially validated drug research in community settings. *Psychopharmacol. Bull.*, 21, 285-90
9. Illich, I. (1975). *Medical Nemesis: the Expropriation of Health*. (London: Calder and Boyers)
10. Robin, R.D. (1984). *Matters of Life and Death: Risks versus Benefits of Medical Care*. (San Francisco: W.H. Freeman)
11. Hartman, D. (1983). The ethics of the patient–doctor relationship: some practical suggestions. *Israel J. Med. Sci.*, 19, 437-41
12. Brinkley, D. (1985). Quality of Life in cancer trials. *Br. Med. J.*, 291, 685-6
13. Joyce, C.R.B. (1985). In Steichele, C., Abshagen, U. and Koch-Weser, J. (eds.). *Drugs between Research and Regulations:* Rauwolfia derivatives and breast cancer: how do we know when we have the answers? (Darmstadt: Steinkopff)
14. Platt, S. (1985). Measuring the burden of psychiatric illness on the family: an evaluation of some rating scales. *Psychol. Med.*, 15, 383-93
15. Fries, J.F. (1983). The assessment of disability: from first to future principles. *Br. J. Rheumatol.*, Supp. 22, 48-58
16. Rosser, R.M. (1983a). Issues of measurement in the design of health indicators: a review. In

Culyer, A.J. (ed.). *Health Indicators* (Oxford: Martin Robertson)

17. Goldberg, D. (1983). Measurement of the benefits in psychiatry. In Teeling-Smith, G. (ed.). *Measuring the Social Benefits of Medicine*, pp. 68–74 (London: Office of Health Economics)

18. Fisch, H.U., Hammond, K.R., Joyce, C.R.B. and O'Reilly, M. (1981). An experimental study of the clinical judgement of general physicians in evaluating and prescribing for depression. *Br. J. Psychiat.*, **138**, 100–9

19. Kirwan, J.R., Chaput de Saintonge, D.M. Joyce, C.R.B. and Currey, H.L.F. (1983). Clinical Judgement Analysis – practical application in rheumatoid arthritis. *Br. J. Rheumatol*, **Supp. 22**, 18–23

20. Hammond, K.R. and Joyce, C.R.B. (eds.). (1975). *Psychoactive Drugs and Social Judgement: Theory and Research.* (New York: John Wiley)

21. Rosser, R.M. (1976). Recent studies using a global approach to measuring illness. *Med. Care,* **15** (Suppl.) No. 5, 138–47

22. Rosser, R. and Kind, P. (1978). A scale of valuations of states of illness; is there a social consensus? *Int. J. Epidemiol.,* **7**, 1347–57

23. Van Raaij, W.F. (1984). Micro and macro economic psychology. *J. Econ. Psychol.,* **5**, 385–401

24. Christensen-Szalanski, J.J.J. (1984). Discount functions and the measurement of patients' values. Women's decisions during childbirth. *Med. Decis. Making*, **4**, 47–58

25. Wenger, N.K., Mattson, M.E., Furberg, C.D. and Elinson, J. (eds.). (1984). *Assessment of Quality of Life in Clinical Trials of Cardiovascular Therapies.* (New York: Le Jacq)

26. Erickson, P., Henke, K.D. and Brittain, R.D. (1983). A health statistics framework: US data systems as a model for European health information? In: Culyer, A.J. (ed.). *Health Indicators*, pp. 117–28 (Oxford: Martin Robertson)

27. Ruberman, W. and Weinblatt, E. (1985). Psychosocial influences on mortality after myocardial infarction. *New Engl. J. Med.*, **312**, 51

28. Sugarbaker, P.H., Barofsky, I., Rosenberg, S.A. and Gionola, F.J. (1982). Quality of life assessment of patients in extremity sarcoma clinical trials. *Surgery*, **91**, 17–23

29. De Haes, J.C.J.M. and van Krippenberg, F.C.E. (1985). The Quality of Life of cancer patients: a review of the literature. *Soc. Sci. Med.*, **20**, 809–17

30. Hunt, S.M., McEwen, J. and McKenna, S.P. (1985). Measuring health status: a new tool for clinicians and epidemiologists. *J. R. Coll. Gen. Pract.*, **35**, 185–8

31. Rosser, R.M. (1983b). A history of the development of health indicators. In Teeling-Smith, G. (ed.). *Measuring the Social Benefits of Medicines*, pp. 50–62. (London: Office of Health Economics)

32. Read, J.L., Quinn, R.J., Berwick, D.M., Fineberg, H.V. and Weinstein, M.C. (1984). Preferences for health outcomes: comparison of assessment methods. *Med. Decis. Making,* **4**, 315–29

33. Culyer, A.J. (1985). A health economist on medical sociology: reflections by an unreconstructed reductionist. *Soc. Sci. Med.*, **20**, 1013–21

Measuring the Benefits of Medicines

Discussion (Chairman: Professor R. Hurley)

PROFESSOR DOLLERY: I felt that the financial arguments put forward by George were fairly specious, because he seemed to imply that financial gain that occurred once could be considered to continue to be taking place forever. As an extreme example, suppose you had abolished tuberculosis; if you then removed all anti-tuberculosis drugs from the market there would be no loss. Even in the areas where he claimed the pharmaceutical industry was making an enormous contribution, it seems the arguments were highly fallible. There is no doubt that overall the pharmaceutical industry has been of benefit to mankind, and that it has been of considerable benefit to the British economy. However, I don't think that it helps anyone to overstate the case as much as he did.

PROFESSOR TEELING SMITH: I do agree that 50% of what Colin said, in that clearly the achievements against tuberculosis are 20 years-old. On the other hand, I find it difficult to see why one is not entitled to talk about those savings. Although they are historical savings, the savings are still real in that if the anti-bacterial drugs had not been developed in the 1950s we would still have queues waiting to get into tuberculosis sanitoria.

In the cost–benefit question, on purely financial terms, it is not possible to take a single snapshot. The £500m or so that the industry in this country is spending on research, and 10 times that world-wide, is not producing medicines for use now but ones that will have their medical impact 15 years ahead. It is equally valid to look back over a similar period and say that the use of the medicine 15 years ago is still producing benefits now. It also seems to be equally valid to take a single point in time and say, for example, that today on the 1st October, the industry saved £Xm as a result of the medicines it produced this morning and a separate account will have to be taken tomorrow. Therefore, I think there is some justification for taking historical savings and setting them against current costs, although I am the first to accept the limitations.

PROFESSOR RAWLINS: No-one in this room would deny the fact that, in mental health, the drugs that have been introduced since the 1950s are wonderful news. On the other hand, you showed data which you actually cannot substantiate. The fact that mental hospitals are empty is partly due to drugs, partly due to changing attitudes, and has been accompanied by the immense cost of community care of patients which you totally ignored.

PROFESSOR TEELING SMITH: That is unfair. If you take, for example, people with mental problems who in the old days would certainly be in mental hospitals, they are now able to make a normal contribution to society, entirely due to modern drugs. I do think that modern medicines in the psychotropic field, which are grossly maligned as being drugs of abuse etc. have made a major contribution.

DR IRVINE: I would like to congratulate Dr Joyce on a splendid and scholarly presentation on an extraordinarily difficult subject and one to which, in this country, we are only beginning to address ourselves with any measure of seriousness. He made an important point in seeking to distinguish between neutral data and the judgements one forms upon them. I wonder if he could say anything further about how patients, that is consumers, might be brought into that process. Insofar as it has gone in this country, we have found it difficult with virtually no mechanisms for enabling that process to happen.

DR JOYCE: Facts are in very short supply, but perhaps I could pinpoint a further difficulty. One of the basic problems in these areas of judgements as a preliminary to action of any kind is to decide by whom these decisions should be made. This is itself a judgement that has to be made. One is, therefore, in a kind of infinite regress, how should we judge who should make the judgements which enable us to then go about the judgements of diagnosis, severity or improvement under therapy, that are the end-subject of interest. For a long time the medical profession made these decisions single-handedly, then there was the phase in which it was recognized to be something to do with the doctor–patient relationship. The pendulum has swung even further now, and there are some people who would say that it is the patient's business. We need a method of deciding what the weights should be that attach to patients, regulators, politicians, physicians etc. I think I know how to do it theoretically, but I am very confused as to how I can do it practically. Perhaps a possible beginning in this country could be made with the General Practice or Patient Advisory Committees. One might, for example, set up a pilot exercise of this kind in a practice with an active, interested group such as this, thereby enabling one to exteriorize what the values and facts are that people are taking into account, what weight they attach to them and how the medical and the lay side can be brought into some kind of approximation to each other by making these things explicit.

DR FITZGERALD: Don't you think we are complicating it. My impression of a good general practitioner is that he mainly encompasses a lot of these skills.

In the classical medical curriculum there is a wide range of sub-specialities, all of which people of a given intellectual capability are expected to master. I am confused as to why we need to say that people who understand bacteriology or physiology cannot understand some other aspect which contains the psycho–social element. Perhaps the reason we are having such a problem is that we have a problem with the emphasis in the medical curriculum. I don't think there is any fundamental reason why a competent doctor cannot handle this particular area of total medical care. I suggest that it is a matter of the educators coming to terms and deciding which things are important. I am not sure that we need to draw in a lot of other activities to flesh out what is basically the doctor's role.

DR JOYCE: I disagree with Desmond Fitzgerald. 300 years ago it was said that 'everyone complains of his memory but no-one complains of his judgements'. While it is perfectly true that doctors ought to be capable of resolving these problems, the fact is that when the items of importance are on the table, even two physicians from the same class in the same medical school will attach different degrees of importance to straightforward things, such as grip strength, morning stiffness and consumption of analgesics in rheumatology. One does need some method of making this more objective than in fact it is.

DR FITZGERALD: I agree about the methodology. The question is who should be applying it? There is a flavour around that another group of people is needed to apply it. I suggest that we should get the educators who teach medical students to bring this much more to the fore. There was a symposium on this subject last year, and a senior registrar attending said all we were talking about was taking a good history. That was an over-simplification, but in a sense it is a large element.

DR CROMIE: Isn't one of the problems that general practitioners, who encompass all these skills, are not treating groups of 100 patients but rather are treating one patient. Their whole practice is to try and maximize the benefit to that individual patient. The individual benefit one requires may be quite different from another one. For example, one patient may not care about his or her grip strength as long as she can get in the morning a bit more easily, while for another patient the most important thing may be to stop any additional medicines because she always forgets to take them. There may be quite different aims for every individual patient, and so the GP is trying to bring all the factors together to give the best quality of life for that patient. This is something which cannot be brought together in a statistical way by someone saying, for example, the overall score is 30%. Perhaps this is one of the difficulties in that all the papers and discussions are concerned with massive groups, whereas doctors are actually treating individual patients.

PROFESSOR WALKER: We are going to try this afternoon to balance benefits and risks, but we have a problem in this session of combining the benefits.

For convenience, we have divided them into clinical, economic and psycho-social, but is there any way in which they can be combined? For example, if one is comparing two similar medicines, how can the clinical, psycho–social and financial benefits be combined into one package?

DR JONES: I think everyone has agreed that if you want to put things together it is necessary to have a common unit, money.

PROFESSOR TEELING SMITH: One of the points that came out of the earlier discussion is the limitation of using money. I believe there are more important things in life than money.

DR JONES: What I meant was that in order to add up three different things it is necessary to reduce them all to a common unit. There is only one we can all agree on, distasteful though it is.

PROFESSOR TEELING SMITH: The chairman raised an important point – we take a very insular view thinking money means something. Our pound is a very unstable currency. I believe that there are more important units, for example quality adjusted life years (QALY). It is an important concept that a year of perfect well-being is worth more than a year of continuous suffering. It is very interesting, looking at the history of health indicators and Rachel Rosser's work, that in the first paper she and her husband Victor Watts presented in 1972, everything had been converted into monetary terms. They had actually used a legal textbook to turn degrees of disability into cash. Subsequently, she moved away, I believe rightly, from that. Money is a misleading unit and we need to think in terms of something broader to measure outcome and well-being.

Session 4

Risk-Benefit Decisions

4.1 Risk–benefit decisions in human administration

Dr R. W. Brimblecombe

It is difficult to estimate risk and it is even more difficult to estimate benefit. One might consider therefore, that is not worth dividing one into the other to produce a risk–benefit ratio which would be impossible to quantify. However, we do live in a real world in which we have to make decisions of risk to benefit and I am going to discuss the world I live in, which is trying to develop new drugs. Specifically I shall talk about the clinical development of drugs, where risk–benefit decisions have to be made rather frequently and regularly.

First the quality, quantity and nature of the information available is different at various points in the drug development process. Second, I would like to re-iterate points already made by Professor Zbinden about the quality of the toxicological animal data available and how we can extrapolate from it.

In considering the information available when making decisions about whether or not to take a drug into man, there are a number of subjective factors to be borne in mind, such as those which follow.

(1) *Proposed Therapeutic Use*
Will the drug be used to treat a life-threatening disease or as a palliative procedure for a trivial condition?

(2) *Expected Duration of Use*
Will it be a one dose situation, or is the drug going to be used for life or for a significant part of it?

(3) *Patient Population*
What will the patient population be -- old, young, etc?

(4) *Availability of Satisfactory Alternatives*
This is an interesting consideration and clearly has to be taken into account by the pharmaceutical company when assessing

whether there will be an available market. However, we should not be obsessed about this, either in the context of marketing or whether or not the drug is taken into man. A great deal has been unexpectedly learned about many drugs simply by taking them into man and observing the results. Many therapeutic indications have been discovered serendipitously by an apparent 'me-too' drug being taken into man with an unexpected and sometimes beneficial finding.

(5)   *Stage of the Development Programme*
Information available to aid these decisions is different at each stage of the development programme as shown in Figure 20. When an initial decision is made whether or not to go into man, the only data available are those derived from animals. Toxicological and pharmacological data are available at that time, and it may be possible, by analogy with drugs that are similar chemically or pharmacologically, to make a guess as to what the drug will or will not do. However, at this stage we are very dependent on the quality, quantity and nature of the non-human data. As we progress through the various stages of clinical testing, the situation changes, although perhaps not in the regular way shown in Figure 20.

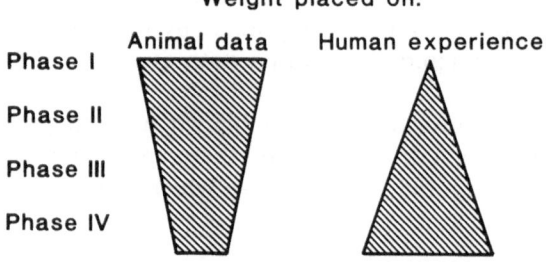

Figure 20 Weight placed on animal and human data at different stages of drug development programme

By the end of Phase I there is at least some clinical experience, although this may not be very helpful from the point of view of safety. It is unusual for florid side-effects to emerge in Phase I studies, presumably because the toxicological data derived from animals have prevented the use of a drug that would produce such effects and have indicated a dose at which it is not likely for serious side-effects to be seen. The important information learned from early human experience relates to metabolic and more particularly pharmacokinetic data. Not many side-effects seen in man have been explainable on the basis of the different metabolism of animals.

On the other hand, many situations in which the animal data are not predictive of what happens in man can be explained on the basis of pharmacokinetic differences. Conversely and paradoxically, an enormous amount of comfort is drawn if it is discovered in the early stage of human experience that the metabolism of the drug in man is indeed similar to what is seen in the species used in the toxicity studies. This also applies to the kinetics.

By the end of Phase I, therefore, some important clinical information is available which provides greater or lesser confidence in the data derived from animals. In addition, by this time more animal data are available. It is normal to go into Phase I studies with perhaps 1 month toxicity in two species and by Phase II results from 3 or 6 months toxicity studies are likely to be available. At Phase III the situation is different again, in that there are still more animal data as the toxicity studies will have run a longer course, and perhaps another species will have been included and so on.

There is one crucial decision point at the beginning of clinical testing, i.e. whether or not to go into man, and there is a second decision point when the marketing stage is reached, i.e. whether or not to apply for marketing authorization. Following marketing, the human experience is much less controlled, in that the drug is not given to selected patients being carefully monitored. This is the most likely situation for unexpected side-effects to turn up. At the point of marketing, the animal data retreat into obscurity. They are not entirely irrelevant by any means, but are much less relevant than they were at the beginning of clinical testing. The human experience comes into full play when the drug is marketed and post-marketing surveillance studies will clearly carry much more weight than everything that has previously taken place. So it is evident that the quality, quantity and nature of the data available varies as there is progression through the stages and certainly becomes dramatically different when marketing is reached.

I would like to return to the information available at the beginning of the clinical programme when the drug is taken into man, either patients or volunteers. These are animal data that allegedly relate to the safety of the drug. No-one should believe that toxicity studies are designed to prove safety – they are conducted to find toxicity. Many of us get very uncomfortable indeed if we don't find toxicity. The purpose of toxicity studies is to detect the target organs and tissues, so that when studies in man are planned particular attention can be paid to the function of these organs and tissues with careful monitoring for adverse effects. Again several factors must be considered, as shown in Table 23.

It is much more important to consider the blood levels achieved rather than the doses applied, although the relationship between the two is often not a simple one. Some knowledge of pharmacokinetics and metabolism

Table 23   Factors to be considered in relation to animal toxicity studies

Doses (blood levels)
Pharmacokinetics
Metabolism
Duration
Frequency of dosing
Findings
     nature
     dose relationship
     no effect level
     one or more species
     mechanisms

is necessary. There are arbitrary rules about the duration of studies which have been carried out in animals in relation to the duration of studies in man. Clearly there is no absolute truth about this, as is evident by the fact that regulations around the world differ markedly. Conventionally, toxicological studies are done by giving the drug once a day, but practically it is not easy to do anything else. Clearly drugs are not always administered once a day and there can be much debate about that.

It is very important to look at the nature of the toxicological findings and to put them into context. We are more impressed by data if there is a relationship between the adverse effect and the dose, and there tends to be an obsession with finding a 'no effect level' in toxicological studies. It is probably worse to see an effect in more than one species, but it is much more important to consider the mechanism of the effect. I strongly suspect that many good drugs have been thrown away unnecessarily simply because people did not take time to look at the mechanism of the effect. I have personal experience of a drug in our own organization which exhibited thyroid toxicity in the rat, but not in the dog or mouse or, from early experience, in man. We discovered that it was increasing the clearance of T-4, resulting in a feedback and stimulation of the thyroid in the rat and was very unlikely to be a hazard for man.

Figure 21 shows the structure of Omeprazole, developed by Astra in Sweden. This is an inhibitor of the 'proton pump' or the hydrogen-

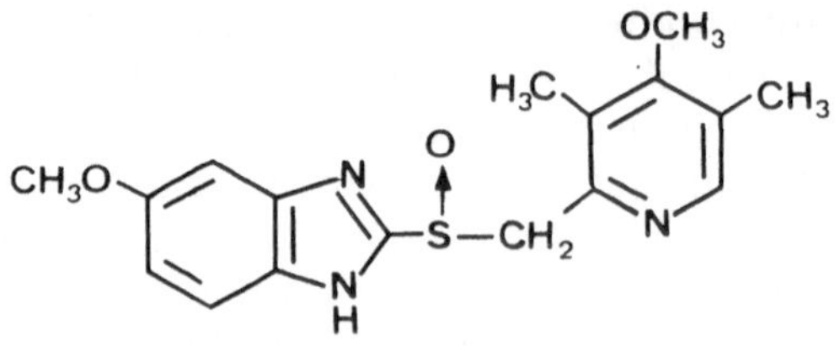

Figure 21   Structure of Omeprazole – an inhibitor of the 'proton pump'

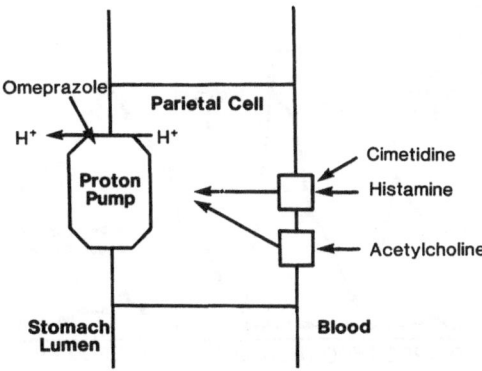

Figure 22 Common pathway of H$^+$ pumping into the stomach

potassium ATPase (Figure 22) which is found in the parietal cells in the stomach. It is the final common pathway in the pumping of hydrogen ions into the stomach. Thus inhibition of the proton pump will inhibit gastric acid secretion. This is a different mechanism to drugs which act as competitive antagonists at either muscarinic receptors or histamine H$_2$ receptors. Drugs like Omeprazole are very effective in reducing gastric acid secretion. Figure 23 shows the effect of Omeprazole in inhibiting histamine-stimulated acid secretion in the Heidenhaim-pouch dog. It is quite clear that it is a potent drug, and very long-acting in comparison to

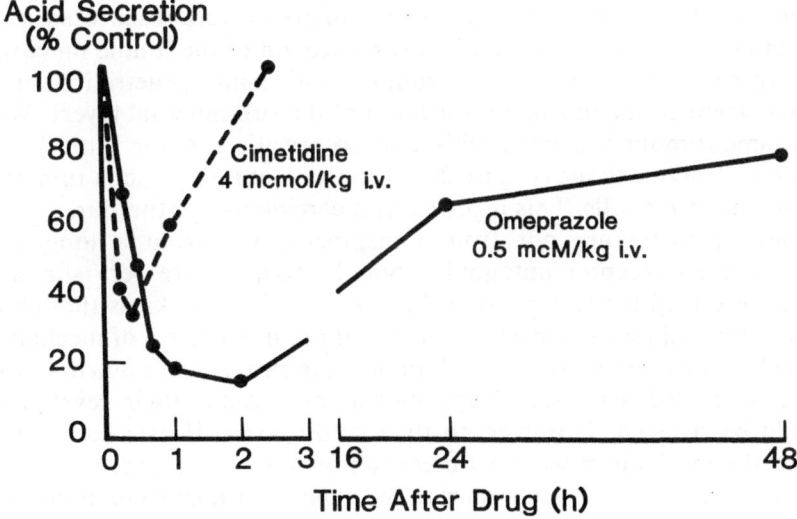

Figure 23 Inhibition of histamine-stimulated acid secretion in the dog

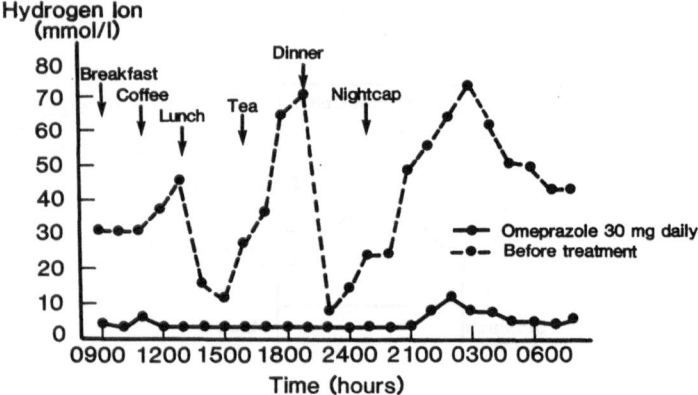

Figure 24   Mean (SEM) hourly intragastric H⁺ activity before and during treatment with Omeprazole 30 mg daily (*n* = 9) (Data from Watt, R.P. *et al.* (1983)

cimetidine. Its effect in the dog is still apparent after 48 hours, while the effect from cimetidine is finished in about 3 hours. It is equally effective in man, as shown in Figure 24. This is a 24 hour study in which hourly intragastric hydrogen ion activity is being measured in an ambulant subject on a normal regime. It can be seen that with 30 mg of Omeprazole daily the subjects are virtually anacidic. This is a very effective drug in healing duodenal ulcer. Trials carried out to date indicate that after 2 weeks treatment with 20–30 mg/day, healing rates of about 90% are achieved for duodenal ulcer. However, tumours were discovered in the rat long-term studies. Figure 25 shows a section of the fundic mucosa of the stomach of rat, showing a tumour with some penetration of the muscular mucosa and some infiltration of the sub-mucosal layers. When this same tumour is stained with a neuro-specific enolase, a marker for neuro-endrocrine tissue (Figure 26), it shows that it is in fact a tumour of neuro-endrocrine cells. This is probably a carcinoid-type tumour.

These pictures are not from Omeprazole but from a long-acting histamine H₂ receptor antagonist, but the pictures are very similar to those described for Omeprazole. In other words, it looks as though any long-acting inhibitor of gastric acid secretion, irrespective of mechanism, is likely to produce these ECL-cell tumours in rats. A while ago one would have concluded that these drugs are carcinogens and their development would be stopped. However, to their credit Astra–Hossle have investigated the mechanism whereby these tumours are produced. The current theory is that these are secondary to the hypergastrinaemia induced by the profound and prolonged anacidity. In human studies, Omeprazole causes small increases in the serum gastrin levels, whereas in toxicity studies in

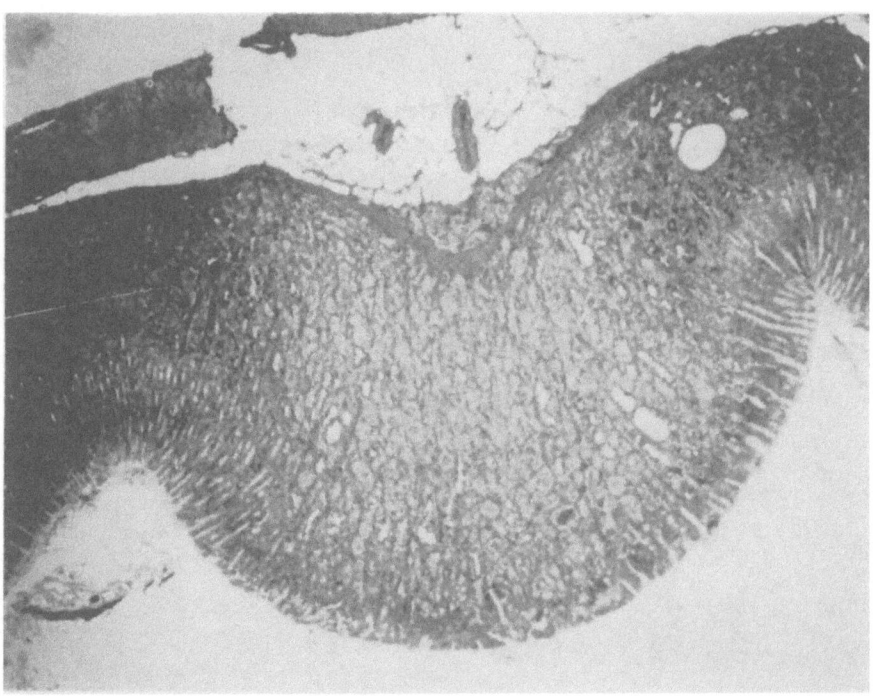

Figure 25   2-year-old rat. Stomach fundic mucosa showing a typical neuro-endocrine tumour with penetration through the muscularis mucosa and infiltration of the submucosa. Haematoxylin and eosin × 60

rats the serum gastrin levels were increased very markedly. It is, therefore, a situation very unlikely to be encountered in the clinic, and may also be specific to the rat (it has not happened in the dog). Omeprazole was withdrawn from clinical trial when these results became available, but it has now been re-instated in at least 10 countries in the world, including Canada and Scandinavia. So this is a situation where the people involved took the trouble to explore the mechanism and have to their satisfaction, and to that of at least some regulatory agencies, decided that this is not an effect which is going to be of any hazard in therapeutic use.

In summary, risk–benefit decisions are extremely difficult as the risk and the benefit are not easily measurable. The data available are in many ways suspect because they often come from the wrong species and drugs are often given to inappropriate numbers at the wrong dose. As this progresses through the development process, the information becomes different, and probably more relevant, so that the decisions taken are based on better information. It is also possible to bring some science into the decisions by exploring the mechanisms of adverse effects when they occur.

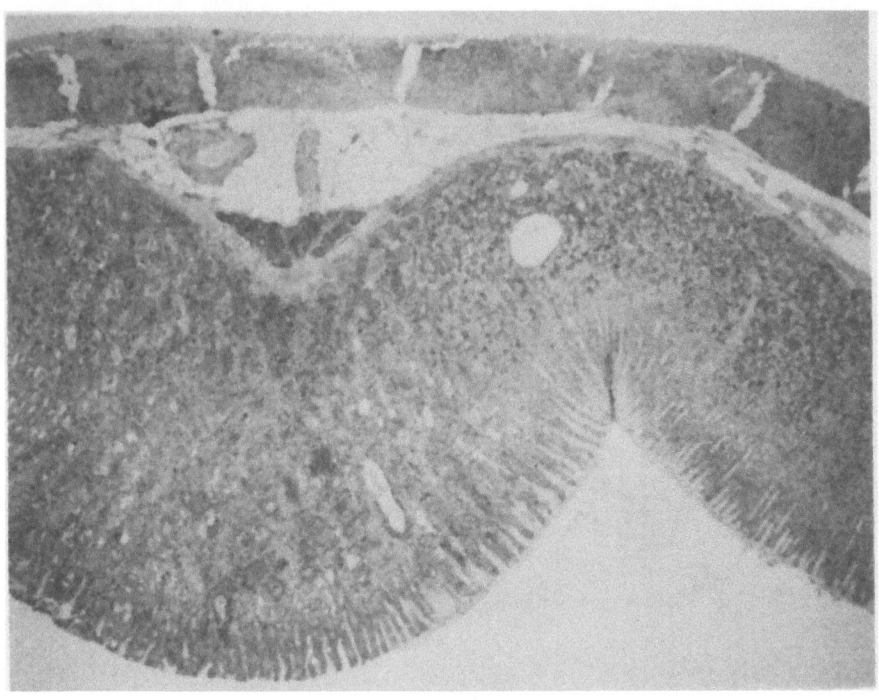

Figure 26   Same tumour stained for neurospecific enolase. (Neurospecific enolase is a marker for neuroendocrine cells). Pap. test × 60

4.1 Risk–benefit decisions in human administration

Discussant: Professor C. F. George

In discussing Dr Brimblecombe's paper, I would like to make the following points.

ATTITUDES OF THE POTENTIAL CLINICAL INVESTIGATOR

The need to develop new chemical entities has at times been questioned. In my view, new drugs are essential for treating diseases that either do not respond at all or in which the existing therapy is unsatisfactory[1]. However, the investigator will attempt to balance the following three elements:

(1) The need for a new drug in a particular disease;
(2) The likelihood of the new compound being an advance over existing treatment;
(3) The possible risks involved.

When the chemical entity is novel, e.g. acyclovir, the justification for further study may be strong. By contrast, the decision to evaluate the umpteenth tricyclic antidepressant, β-adrenoceptor antagonist or non-steroidal anti-inflammatory drug may be more difficult. In my view, the compound should offer a potential advantage over its predecessors. Such an advantage might be a greater selectivity for a particular receptor type – thus reducing the potential for side-effects. Alternatively, it could be easier to use by virtue of a longer duration of action, improved absorption characteristics or reduced pre-systemic metabolism. However, assessment of the likely risks involved may be easier when one is studying analogues of existing compounds which have already been introduced into clinical practice rather than with novel substances.

Nevertheless, assessment of the potential risks is inevitably something of a gamble. Although pre-clinical toxicity testing is both necessary and can identify potential problems, it can have no absolute predictive value for unwanted effects in man. Professor Dollery has already alluded to the fact that CNS effects may be easier to detect in man. In this context, I would cite studies which we undertook of a new imidazoline drug. These totalled only five and were performed in two individuals. Despite the fact that increased cardiac contractility occurred, it was decided to abandon the investigations at a very early stage because of the occurrence of xanthopsia during the intravenous infusion of this drug. No amount of animal toxicity testing would have predicted this effect, since you can't talk to a rat!

One other important point concerning pre-clinical toxicity data is that the clinical investigator should not proceed unless he is satisfied that these are adequate. He should resolve any doubts that he has by personal discussion with the pharmacologist concerned and/or an independent expert(s)[2].

RESEARCH IN HUMANS

It is important to remember that evaluation of new chemical entities in humans carries several different risks. The first of these is the risk of the procedure itself, e.g. arterial cannulation or the infusion of substances intravascularly. These should be very small, provided that such procedures are carried out in a well equipped laboratory by competent and experienced staff. Second, there are the risks of inadequate care which may relate both to the nature of the research and where this is being carried out. Syncope is by far the most common adverse consequence of a procedure and may, rarely, be of sufficient severity to require resuscitation of the healthy volunteer or patient. Unexpected or unforeseen events may occur despite care taken in both planning and execution of drug studies in man. Human subjects require the highest standards of medical care if they should fall ill during the course of an investigation.

When healthy volunteers are being studied, it is important that they are screened carefully for previously occult disease. Furthermore, it may be necessary to test them for the presence of other drug substances, particularly those of abuse. The third possibility (and the least likely) is an adverse effect from the drug itself. By far the most common is a true side-effect relating to the drug's main pharmacological action. Such problems which include hypotension from an α-adrenoceptor blocking drug, tachycardia from the administration of a β-adrenoceptor stimulant or unpleasant CNS symptoms due to a dopamine receptor blocking drug can usually be predicted. Furthermore, they can be minimized with appropriate care in the design of the experiment: well-trained staff should have no difficulty in coping with them. Type B reactions are a matter of great concern in human drug studies. Experience would indicate that they are comparatively rare, but they are more likely to occur when high or repeated doses are given. Appropriate assessment of organ function in man (based upon experience in the pre-clinical toxicity studies) should be an adequate safeguard. However, in my view there is no justification for so-called 'human tolerance' studies being conducted in healthy volunteers.

CONCLUSIONS

There is a need for new medicines, especially for diseases that do not respond at all to known medication, but also for others in which the existing treatment is unsatisfactory. Provided that studies in man are carefully planned and executed in appropriate surroundings, the hazards of administering new chemical entities to man are small. My experience is mirrored by that of my colleagues in clinical pharmacology and by that within the pharmaceutical industry (Griffin (1985), personal communication).

References

1. George, C.F. (1981). The importance of clinical pharmacology in drug development. *Clin. Sci.* **60**, 247–50
2. Laurence, D.R. (1961). Discussion of the transfer of drugs from the animal laboratory to man. *Proc. R. Soc. Med.*, **54**, 206

4.2 Risk–benefit decisions in product licence applications

Professor R. Bass

The papers presented have demonstrated that the licensing of a drug is a permanent process. Although the granting of a licence – or not – is a very important time in the life of a drug, risk–benefit decisions are also made before and after this event. They are made early on in the development by the pharmaceutical manufacturer, then at the Investigational New Drug (IND) and New Drug Application (NDA) stage by the pharmaceutical manufacturer and the regulatory agency concerned, the later on also by the physician. Whenever new data are available, an update of the risk–benefit decision is required. The evaluation carried out can change the balance from good to bad or vice versa.

It is our task to describe the role that regulatory agencies play in this process. This influence could be explained best (and it would be most interesting to all of us) if problematic cases of risk–benefit decisions concerning the pre-marketing stage were discussed. Since this is not possible, this paper will begin with a general description of how the feeding of the decision wheel with new data works. This will be followed by a description of the process of making some actual risk–benefit decisions that have led to marketing authorization in some countries, while in other countries authorization was refused, is still pending, or was superseded by removal from the market. The situations described are, however, similar in all other stages of drug development. Thus we can obtain indirect information on how decisions are reached at the regulatory agency during the pre-marketing stage.

SOME GENERAL REMARKS ON RISK-BENEFIT DECISIONS

Generally speaking risk–benefit decisions are based on legislation which is comparable throughout the western world. Different outcomes of

127

decisions in different countries depend on the details of the individual case. The difference can be based on differences in administrative and scientific views and interpretation. Quite often it is the difference in the time at which a decision is made which leads to deviating opinions. Questions which arise later can delay the marketing of a drug, lead to a restriction in proposed use, change approved labelling or prevent introduction altogether.

Final conclusions should not, if possible, be drawn from a single source of data or from the outcome of a single study. Pharmaceutical manufacturers and regulatory agencies must always attempt to gather all the important information available on pharmacology, pharmacokinetics, exposure and clinical studies, and thence judge the validity of the data. Furthermore, the substance being evaluated must be compared with the available alternatives (benefit–benefit and risk–risk evaluation). This is particularly true when there is a large number of chemically-related alternatives with a large range of irreversible toxic effects such as carcinogenicity, teratogenicity, liver cirrhosis, etc., or toxic effects which unmask themselves only after long periods or several generations, such as mutagenicity at the germ cell level.

We cannot ignore the fact that decisions must often be made on the basis of incomplete data. Decisions are made as a series of incremental steps on the basis of the data available at the time of the decision. This assumes the impossibility of everlasting 'correct' decisions and implies international deviations. Often a theoretical evaluation based on data from animal experiments is superseded by a more practical evaluation based on clinical practice. The pharmaceutical industry has made re-evaluation such a standard procedure that even the half-life for the marketing phase of a drug have been calculated, i.e., the time at which the 'old' drug must be replaced by a 'new' drug. Such 'Standard Operating Procedures' cannot influence the decision of the regulatory agency.

EXAMPLES OF RISK–BENEFIT DECISIONS

Interestingly enough all the cases I shall describe deal with problems of carcinogenicity or carcinogenic potential. This unwanted effect is suspected from, or detected in, short-term studies or long-term animal experiments and, therefore, can turn up at any time during development. The data mentioned here are already known or are available to the public. Of course it is true that quantification of a carcinogenic risk for man is still quite impossible. We circumvent, or mask, this problem by talking about risk–benefit decisions, thus admitting the great relativity, which is influenced both by society (social acceptance of risks) and by technology (feasible safety measures). It is usually impossible to sufficiently handle risk, especially carcinogenic risk, at the post-marketing stage by applying data from long-term use in man. It, therefore, seems necessary to reach risk–benefit decisions by employing data from animal experiments, taking into account all other information available. In order to avoid indication of our personal likes and dislikes, I shall discuss the products in the order that the applications were filed.

Molsidomin

This is a drug used in the treatment of angina pectoris and some specific forms of cardiac failure. It was first marketed in Japan in 1972 and later on in Germany and other countries. At the end of 1981, we received information that chronic toxicity and carcinogenicity studies had revealed a carcinogenic potential: tumours were seen in the nose of rats at 50 ppm (3mg/kg, approximately 30 times the dose given to man), 320 ppm and 2000 ppm in the powdered diet.

At that time it was argued that application of molsidomin in the powdered diet – in contrast to the addition of molsidomin in the drinking water in the earlier Japanese negative studies – could have led to local damage and chronic inflammation in the nose, or that the effect was partly due to the diet or the bedding. Although the risk–benefit decision remained positive, our hesitance in accepting such an explanation led to a request for further investigation. In the carcinogenicity study then performed, the effects of molsidomin given at approximately 1000 ppm in the drinking water or in the powdered diet were compared in all groups. After the results of this study became available in 1985, the Federal Health Office decided to suspend the licence, pending further classification of the carcinogenic effects observed. The risk–benefit decision at that time was negative, although extrapolation of the effects observed in rats to man had not yet been possible.

The histo-pathological investigation of the nasal areas revealed two types of reactions:

(1)   Independent of the mode of application of molsidomin and of the type of diet fed to the animals, including controls, inflammatory processes occurred and were pronounced in the apical region of the nose. Plant or starch particles found in this region make it likely that these reactions were due to such particles. Even without molsidomin application, the inflamed areas showed hyperplasia and metaplasia. Inflammation was observed after as little as 6 months. Areas of acute inflammation showed necrosis and large ulcerations. Chronic alterations often showed apparently normal epithelium. There were no tumours in these

areas and the same changes were seen in all groups.

(2)   Many of the treated animals showed adenomous proliferations of the nasal mucous membranes, oriented towards the ethmoid, in regions devoid of inflammation. Solitary and multicentric localizations were both apparent, the size varying from small ones to nodules giving the appearance of adenomatas. In some cases invasive growth and signs of undifferentiated carcinoma were seen. Furthermore, in all groups approximate equal numbers of undifferentiated carcinoma (25%) were observed and sub-classification was possible. Since, although chronic inflammation occurred in all groups, tumours were seen only in treated animals and, furthermore, since tumours occurred in uninflamed areas, it was concluded that molsidomin was the cause of the tumours.

Understanding and classifying the carcinogenic potential of molsidomin from the data obtained in rats proved problematic. Its metabolism gave no clear-cut indication of the occurrence of possible nitroso-compounds. A rat-specific pattern of metabolites could not be found, nose and liver carry, qualitatively, the same metabolites. In many mutagenicity studies negative results were obtained. These data would have been judged adequate to sufficiently rule out a mutagenic action of the compound in man were it not for the suspicion of a carcinogenic potential. This rendered the data base insufficient for exclusion of the possibility of a genotoxic mechanism of action for the development of tumours. For the metabolite Sin I, positive as well as negative data are available from mutagenicity studies. Whereas gene mutation tests with *Escherichia coli* showed no mutations, *Salmonella typhimurium* (Ames test) yielded reproducible positive results at doses well below cytotoxicity. UDS-tests (with embryonal hamster fibroblasts and human fibroblasts) showed weak positive results at doses close to those leading to cytotoxicity. One micronucleus test (mouse) was negative, but it was not performed according to modern scientific requirements. From these data a mutagenic potential has to be suspected for Sin I. The effects observed were discussed as being due to spontaneous denitrosation, possibly leading to nitrite concentrations high enough to allow mutagenicity. Sin Ic is the only other metabolite investigated. A study with *S. typhimurium* (Ames test) yielded marginal positive results in the presence of an activation system. The results were discussed as weak and were unable to explain the positive results with the prior metabolite, Sin I. Overall, the results from mutagenicity studies do not sufficiently rule out the possibility of an underlying genotoxic action for the carcinogenic effects observed.

The data and these evaluations were presented at a public hearing in December 1985 in Berlin (the German Drug Act requires hearings to be held before severe changes of the marketing status of a drug can be permanently enacted). At the hearing, it was agreed that the 'justified' suspicion that led to the temporary suspension of the marketing licence did exist. However, specific indications for use, e.g. for the treatment of cases of angina pectoris and myocardial infarction in which nitrates were ineffective or not tolerated or in which reduced coronary flow was present, were also presented. These were substantiated by clinical trials and reports of experience. The risk–benefit assessment for the use of molsidomin for these indications was then compared to those of available alternatives.

The weight of scientific evidence is in favour of the assumption that the mutagenic action of molsidomin is hypothetical. At present existing data provide no sufficient evidence to substantiate a mutagenic action. Therefore, by conventional definition there is a tendency towards classifying the risk–benefit decision again as being positive, thereby allowing the use of molsidomin, but only for defined cases of angina pectoris and of myocardial infarction.

For a regulatory agency, this process of first suspending and then re-granting a licence is a normal process. The molsidomin case has been described here in some detail in order to demonstrate that suspension does not necessarily always lead to permanent revocation. The temporary removal from the market serves the purpose of clarifying the issue. After clarification the product may then be replaced on the market with new conditions.

Isosorbide-5-mono-nitrate and isosorbide-di-nitrate

Isosorbide-5-mono-nitrate was classified a new drug in Germany. Because of this and the indications claimed, carcinogenicity studies were required. On the basis of clinical experience with isosorbide-di-nitrate, a licence for isosorbide-5-mono-nitrate was granted with the condition that such a study be initiated immediately. During the last year the clinical use of isosorbide-di-nitrate has changed drastically; the doses used have been increased to more than 100 mg/day. Thus clinical experience could no longer be cited as proof of the lack of a carcinogenic effect. The need for such studies was also pointed out by some mutagenicity data and the glyceryl trinitrate study of the USA army. The required investigation is now well under way as a joint venture by most companies concerned. They were linked up by the German Pharmaceutical Manufacturers Association (BPI). Interim results after 2 years indicate no carcinogenic potential. The risk–benefit decision remains positive for the time being.

Budesonide

Budesonide is a steroidal antiphlogistic agent with little systemic action. It is used by inhalation for asthma, and on the skin. Products containing this substance have been on the market in Germany for several years. For such compounds one used to be very hesitant to perform or ask for carcinogenicity studies. We received the data of a rat carcinogenicity study (Sprague–Dawley CR/CD strain from Charles River Inc.) showing an increase in astrocytomas at the highest dose used ($50\mu g kg^{-1}$ day^{-1}), tumours occurred in males only. The other doses were 0, 10 and $25\mu g kg^{-1}$ day^{-1}. A great deal of discussion has been going on about the types of tumours, their size, localization and so on. Overall, it is likely that these tumours are of the same kind as tumours seen in controls. The frequency of this tumour varies greatly in various control groups and strains.

The evidence is, however, insufficient to prove or disprove that in the case of budesonide we are dealing with a chance result. It seems possible that there is a substance-related, possibly neurocarcinogenic action. There were no tumours in females, none in mice, and no other relevant tumour localizations in the nervous system or other organs. Most tumours were small and appeared late. There were no signs of either pre-neoplastic changes or malignancy. Histological comparison showed no differences between gliomas in controls and in treated groups. There were no obvious signs of immunosuppression. Nevertheless, the tumours might be due to hormonal action leading to excess glial proliferation. In the rat, the persisting activity of the subependymic matrix of the glial cells makes this possible during the whole lifespan. In man, the proliferative capacity of glial cells ceases physiologically soon after birth.

Mutagenicity studies gave negative results. On the basis of this evidence, the risk–benefit decision remained positive and budesonide was left on the market. This drug and its carcinogenic potential was also discussed with a similar conclusion at the Safety Working Party of the Committee of Proprietary Medicinal Products (CPMP).

To further clarify the issue, new carcinogenicity studies have been required and are under way. A comparison with other steroidal antiphlogistics has yielded no helpful conclusions.

Indoprofen

Indoprofen is a non-steroidal anti-inflammatory agent. In rats, dose-dependently induced tumours of the intestine were produced. There were chronic ulcerations with pronounced fibrosation, chronic ulcerations with adenoma–carcinoma and well-differentiated and undifferentiated adeno-carcinoma not apparently connected to ulcerations.

In control rats ulcus-carcinoma occur only very rarely. Under similar conditions, i.e. in doses and duration of treatment relatively the same as the doses and duration of treatment given to man, 18 other non-steroidals did not lead to intestinal carcinoma in rats, even though a high frequency of ulceration was observed for all of them. It has been proposed that the effects seen with indoprofen are due to its special pharmacokinetic behaviour: enterohepatic recirculation yields very high local concentrations.

In order to gain time to clarify the issue of tumour risk as well as that of clinically observed adverse reactions, the licence for indoprofen was suspended some time ago. In the meantime the company that had marketed indoprofen in the Federal Republic of Germany has waived its claim for the licence. A positive or negative risk–benefit decision had not yet been reached at our agency at that point of time.

Brotizolam

Brotizolam is a benzodiazepine-related hypnotic agent. This compound has also been reviewed by the Safety Working Party of the CPMP. Despite continuing suspicions of a carcinogenic potential, this Working Party recommended marketing authorization or maintenance of the current status of brotizolam containing drugs in the member states.

The suspicion of carcinogenic potential is based on an increased rate of neurilemmomas of the rat uterus. These may be interpreted as 'false-positives', or as an indication of a carcinogenic potential. Even assuming a carcinogenic potential, the following points influence interpretation towards a more positive risk–benefit evaluation:

(1) A carcinogenicity study in mice gave no indication for carcinogenic potential;

(2) A chronic toxicity study in rats for 18 months did not yield an increased tumour rate;

(3) There is no indication of a genotoxic potential of brotizolam;

(4) With brotizolam the highest dose tested exceeded the therapeutic dose by 100 times (and the same holds true when looking at serum concentrations) even though the recommended high dose is not required to exceed the therapeutic dose by 100 times;

(5) Neurilemmomas occur under brotizolam close to, or within, the frequency range shown by 'historical controls' for this type of tumour;

(6) The rat is metabolically quite different from man and mouse.

CONCLUSION

We hope that we have been able to demonstrate the diversity of risk–benefit decisions stemming from questions regarding a carcinogenic potential of drugs.

We have to be aware of the present situation, i.e. of varying standards of evaluation in the various countries, which complicate the issue.

Our experience with the EEC, CPMP and Safety Working Party has shown that fruitful discussions can help to clarify issues. Varying stages of marketing in various countries, however, will remain a major source of varying risk–benefit decisions in the countries concerned.

Decisions made until now were almost never based on quantitative data. Because risk–benefit decisions usually cannot wait until conclusive quantitative data have been generated, they are subject to revision when such information becomes available.

Acknowledgement

The author wishes to associate the names of Volker Schmidt, Stephen Madle and Roger Grase with this paper.

4.2 Risk–benefit decisions in product licence applications

Discussant: Dr B. W. Cromie

Professor Bass has presented some very interesting case reports, and I shall now discuss some of the principles involved. There are many people in this audience who have served either on the Medicines Commission or the Section 4 Committees, and everyone involved has had three words impressed upon their minds: quality, safety and efficacy. These are the three guidelines for giving product licences by the licensing authority, who looks at risk with respect to safety and quality and at risk–benefit with respect to efficacy. We all realize that the licensing authority has to make decisions, both on risk–benefit ratios and on whether a product should be marketed, with very limited knowledge. We, therefore, understand how difficult the task is for the CSM and the other committees, when they have limited knowledge; not very many patients and animal data which may or may not be relevant. One of the other problems which the licensing authority has is that medicine, in this country, is effectively an individual business, in that the doctor is treating one patient and trying to assess risk–benefit for him. The licensing authority has to look at group results and, therefore, sometimes tends to forget risk and benefits which may be applicable to an individual, so that benefits to a minority group can become lost.

In recent years, the licensing authority has taken an active role, not only in refusing licences, but in reviewing them later. We have seen how Butazolidin and Tanderil have been withdrawn. This means that the licensing authority is extending its responsibility for safety and efficacy and is keeping a 'watching brief' for all medicines throughout their lives. Drugs are removed from the market which, although theoretically more harmful, are often the ones which people were familiar with. This could well be more dangerous than letting them remain on the market as, if familiar drugs are withdrawn, doctors are forced to use other drugs which they know less well.

Having had the three words, safety, quality and efficacy, imprinted on

135

our minds, the government, rather than the licensing authority, have now taken a complete reverse turn. First of all they seem to be allowing medicines to be imported where the quality is uncertain. More important is their action on the Limited List, where they have actively banned medicines which were found to be safe and effective. Trial and error is very important in finding out what is the best medicine for an individual patient, and removing products completely is a very significant move in which the government is taking an even greater degree of responsibility in directing the way in which doctors use their medicines. Already with benzodiazepines, which is a slightly controversial area, there is some evidence that doctors have been pushed to use more potent and potentially more dangerous benzodiazepines in place of the ones that have been removed. Therefore the risk–benefit ratio is being altered by the action of the government, albeit not, in this case, the licensing authority.

Licensing authorities have a difficult task already, but one new factor which may make it even more difficult is the EEC Directive which has just been passed on strict liability. This country, as a signatory, will eventually have to incorporate this into its law. The UK is likely to modify the strict liability by including the 'state of the art' defence, but I suspect this defence will eventually be lost. If the risk–benefit ratio goes in the wrong direction and there is a greater risk than expected, who is responsible? Is it the manufacturer or is it the licensing authority who has, to a large extent, decided on the programme of testing and eventually given the permission to market? This new legislation, where clearly there must be a shared responsibility between manufacturers and licensing authority, will concentrate minds and perhaps make life even more difficult for the licensing authority as well as for the pharmaceutical industry. It might also persuade government on the need for a government 'safety-net' as part of an insurance package to cope with strict liability for medicines.

I suspect that one of the factors in all of this is that to achieve decent laws it is necessary to persuade the public, who persuade the media who persuade the politicians. Eventually an understanding amongst people generally is reached. All of us have shown, however, that it is almost impossible to put across the benefit side. We have an enormous problem as a licensing authority and as an industry to get the risk–benefit understanding through to the general population. Personally I have tried to interest television producers in putting on programmes to get a balanced view of risk–benefit, but they are just not concerned. Perhaps the new strict liability law may make patients, with the help of some lawyers, a little more understanding of their rights, or their perceived rights, when things go wrong. It may make them begin to understand risk and benefit in a better or clearer way. So this law may affect us all, and in the end make the risk–benefit ratio something everyone will have to look at in a different way.

4.3 Risk–benefit decisions in licensing changes

Professor M. D. Rawlins

At the time drugs are licensed evidence for the efficacy and safety of a new compound will have been more or less secured. At this stage, efficacy has often only been established in a limited number of patients under a narrow range of conditions, and safety in relatively small numbers for a short duration. During the post-marketing period, evidence may accumulate to suggest that the efficacy is considerable in a wider group of patients than was originally indicated, and that safety during long-term use in a more heterogeneous population is acceptable. Alternatively, efficacy may appear to be less satisfactory than originally believed and safety becomes prejudiced. The good news is relatively easy to evaluate, and I am going to concentrate on the bad news which is much more difficult to assess. My paper will, therefore, address risk–benefit assessment when there is an apparent problem.

Firstly I would like to consider the issues that are not discussed in licensing changes, subsequently those which are considered, and finally consider how a risk–benefit assessment is achieved. The views presented are not necessarily those of the Committee, but rather those of an individual who has served on the CSM for a number of years.

There are certain issues that, contrary to what people say and believe, are not actually considered in licensing changes. These are shown in Table 24.

Firstly, the financial impact on the company is not considered. On one occasion it was suggested that an adverse decision would have an adverse impact on a particular company's financial position, but that suggestion did not come from the company concerned. It has also been erroneously suggested that members of the Committee on Safety of Medicines might be influenced by the contact they have with competitors or the company under consideration.

With regard to unknown and unsuspected benefits, it has been suggested that these should be taken into consideration. Unfortunately,

Table 24   Issues *not* considered by the CSM

(1)   Impact on company/competitors
(2)   Unknown/unsuspected benefits (e.g. zomepirac)
(3)   Decisions by other regulatory authorities

(4)   Misuse
    (a) Potential (e.g. cannabinoids)
    (b) Actual (e.g. paracetamol, dextropropoxyphene)

(5)   Pressure
    (a) Parliament (e.g. Debendox, Depo-Provera)
    (b) Media
    (c) Pressure Groups (e.g. Reye's syndrome and Valproate)

when members of the CSM are invited to serve, they are not issued with crystal balls enabling them to gaze into the future.

The third issue that is not considered are decisions made by other regulatory authorities. The evidence upon which they have made their decision, if in fact there is any, may be considered. However, in my experience the CSM has not decided on an issue because the BGA, the FDA, or the Swedish authority has taken a particular decision.

The fourth issue that is not generally considered is the potential or actual misuse of drugs by patients. There have been suggestions in the recent past that certain drugs should be removed from the market, for example cannabinoids, because of their potential for causing cannabis-like highs, or dextropropoxyphene-containing products, because of the high risk from over-dosage. The misuse of drugs other than in the stated indications is not taken into account.

Finally, the CSM is often accused of allowing itself to be pressurized into making decisions by Parliament, by the media and by pressure groups. It has been suggested that, in response to hostile parliamentary questions or 'Early Day Motions', the CSM will make decisions based on what certain Members of Parliament want that morning. It is also thought that a number of journalists can influence the CSM or that pressure groups can influence a decision one way or another. Pressure will make the CSM look at issues; pressure does not enter into the final decision. Examples of this include Debendox, where over a number of years there was immense pressure from Parliament, the media and from lay pressure groups to withdraw it on the grounds of teratogenicity. The CSM examined the issue on many occasions in response to that pressure, but at no time did it recommend withdrawal. Similarly, with Depo-Provera, the CSM was pressed never to license it, nor to enlarge its indications and also to withdraw it. However, in fact Depo-Provera remains available on the market with its licensed indication for long-term contraception. Pressures on the Committee to withdraw Valproate is another example. Pressure does make the Committee look at problems, but it does not make the Committee take a licensing action unless it feels there are positive reasons for doing so.

The positive issues that are considered as a basis for licensing action are written in tablets of stone in the Medicines Act: Quality, Efficacy and Safety, as shown in Table 25.

Quality is not usually a problem for licensing changes; if there is a

Table 25   Issues considered by the CSM

(1)   Quality
(2)   Efficacy
     (a) New evidence for lack of efficacy
     (b) Uniqueness of therapeutic properties
     (c) Uniqueness of efficacy in small patient subgroups
(3)   Safety
     (a) Spontaneous reports
         –literature
         –yellow cards
         –other agencies
     (b) Cohort studies
     (c) Case-control studies
     (d) Animal carcinogenicity

quality issue the licensing authority usually takes rapid action. The common problem results when there is an apparent safety issue with a licensed product. When this occurs, it is critical to examine the evidence both for efficacy and for safety. When examining this evidence, the CSM looks first of all at the uniqueness of the therapeutic properties of the particular compound. In addition, a common plea of pharmaceutical companies, particularly when there is a problem with one of their drugs, is that a compound has unique efficacy in a small patient sub-group. A major difficulty arises in deciding whether this is the case, as often there is no formal evidence and the CSM must rely on the testimony of individual specialists in the particular discipline.

In evaluating safety, information from a variety of sources is available. Spontaneous reports, both in the worldwide literature and through the British yellow card reporting system, are particularly important. If licensing action is contemplated against a particular drug, the yellow cards are individually scrutinized to ensure that there have been no coding problems, no double counting, and so that the medical assessor can then re-evaluate the strength of the association between administration of the drug and the suspected adverse effect in individual cases. This individual scrutiny often involves not only the drug under consideration, but also other drugs within a similar therapeutic class. The numbers of yellow cards are looked at in relation to the number of prescriptions for the drug, and there are many confounding factors which are always present in the Committee's mind. The life of the product, the marketing claims, whether the compound has had media attention and, more recently, whether the drug has been subject to post-marketing surveillance as this may influence the number of spontaneous reports, are all considered. The yellow card prescription related adverse reactions may be examined in comparison with other members of the same therapeutic class. Sometimes this highlights disparities, for example the number of cases of Guillain–Barré syndrome appearing in association with Zimelidine, in relation to the number of prescriptions and other reports of peripheral neuropathy, was examined and these greatly exceeded any other marketed antidepressant. On occasions we also have available adverse reaction reports from other agencies, although the British yellow card system is probably as good as any other in the world. However, if information is available, for example from the Swedish regulatory authority, that too may be examined by the Committee.

Other safety data that may be available include case control or cohort studies, sometimes published in the literature and very often carried out by the company and available in company reports. In addition, and in many ways causing more intellectual problems than most others, positive animal carcinogenicity results may occasionally be reported for a marketed compound. We have already discussed extrapolation of animal data to predict human adverse reactions. Great difficulty arises when dealing with an established drug that has been available for many years if, on the one hand there is a lack of adverse reaction reports or epidemiological evidence to show an association between a cancer and the drug. However, on the other hand, one knows that such an association, particularly with common tumours, may well have been missed.

That brings us to risk–benefit assessment and how this is carried out. My observation is that a risk–benefit assessment for licensing change is carried out in the same way as other regulatory authorities dealing with such issues. There are basically three methods: (1) formal analysis, (2) comparative analysis, and (3) judgement.

Firstly, formal analysis or cost–benefit analysis. The problems with this have already been clearly enunciated by Colin Dollery; it is the problem of comparing apples and pears, or of titrating one life saved versus 1000 patients with impotence. Occasionally formal analysis is possible. For example, this has been done with oral contraceptives where lives lost versus lives saved falls heavily in the balance of the latter. However, it is very unusual in my experience for formal analysis to be particularly helpful.

The second approach is the comparative method, or what the Americans call 'boot-strapping'. A particular drug is compared with similar drugs and if the risks and benefits appear to be similar, then the drug is allowed to remain on the market. This is probably a very common way in which evaluations have been made. The great risk, however, is that one may be caught out with time, since what constituted a satisfactory risk–benefit assessment 20 or 30 years ago may not represent a satisfactory assessment now. In fact, when it comes to pharmaceuticals there are relatively small numbers of drugs for which such a comparative estimate can be made.

In truth, the majority of risk–benefit decisions are made on a judgemental basis. The people who make individual decisions are subject to biases; some will be risk-prone while others will be risk-averse on a particular issue. Experts, as we know, are fallible. Other groups might well reach different decisions on another occasion, even when presented with the same data. Indeed, I sometimes wonder if we ourselves would make the same decision on another occasion when presented with the same data.

Thus regulatory authorities have relatively crude tools with which to make decisions on licensing drugs. We are sometimes uncertain of the evidence of efficacy, there is often incomplete definition of the hazard and a poor estimate of the risk. Invariably risk–benefit assessment is based on the fallibility of human judgement.

4.3 Risk-benefit decisions in licensing changes

Discussant: Dr D. Irvine

It is at this point that the fallibility of human judgement enters in, for as a clinician I start with patients, where the regulatory body leaves off. Mike Rawlins described it as a relatively crude mechanism for sifting and sorting the process of defining benefits and risks, but it is nevertheless important. As a practising clinician, I take information from the regulatory body and from other sources in seeking practical and up-to-date guidance on such matters as quality, efficacy and, in particular, safety. As a family doctor I spend a large part of my time prescribing. I work at two different levels; firstly by tradition at the personal level with individual patients, who are, or think they are, ill, and secondly with those patients who are well but want a service which may include giving a drug, for example vaccination, or antenatal care. A third dimension has entered into my field of work only relatively recently, that is anticipatory care where I or my team go out to search for vulnerable groups in the population who may be at risk, for example from suspected blood pressure or diabetes. This adds a new dimension to the risk-benefit question.

At the individual level, as a doctor I rely on being kept up-to-date with good information about the safety and reliability of drugs. Considerable improvements in the availability of such information have been made, not least through the efforts of the CSM itself. There is also the additional fact that doctors are becoming more conscious of their responsibilities as prescribers in all dimensions.

When the patient comes to the consulting room the 'fine-tuning' begins, where the exercise of my judgement is invariably combined with that of the patient's. Sometimes the decisions are easy and obvious, such as whether to prescribe or not, and what to prescribe. I have found, even in the last year or two, how much more conscious I have become about questions of prescribing, in particular whether to prescribe at all. Even more so, my patients who are ordinary working people, are themselves interested in what I might or might not prescribe. Often the statements, 'You are not going to prescribe for me, are you doctor?' or 'Do I really need a drug?' will come from a patient, particularly a woman who is pregnant. The opening statement may also be, after we have established pregnancy, 'I don't want a drug'. This is all relatively recent and is engendered largely by the discussions in the media which have had a profound effect.

The media, however, is only one source in this wider issue. Patients' perceptions are not always what they seem. What we, as doctors, often think are good for our patients are not what our patients actually want themselves. In particular, it is very interesting to see that as the risk of death may be relatively remote for the individual person, they find the notion of mortality difficult to grasp, whereas the concept of morbidity is not. Many of my discussions are concerned with the relative benefits to be drawn from a particular drug weighed against possible hazards or uncomfortable side-effects.

An example of this dilemma is to be found in patients with rheumatoid arthritis, where the question of dyspeptic symptoms or the irritation of a duodenal ulcer must be matched against the patient's requirement for comfort. There is more often than not a negotiation or discussion which can lead to different outcomes in different individuals. This is where the 'fine tuning' element comes in. In the limited list controversy, it has been my experience that a small number of patients who needed analgesic drugs, particularly for chronic rheumatic conditions, who had themselves exercised the fine tuning, have noted the loss of it by the removal of those drugs from the market. It is interesting that we have had to devise methods of introducing new generics. Co-codamol effervescent BP always gets paracodol because paracodol worked for a lot of patients. This leaves the scientists gasping and horror-struck, but leaves at least a small minority of patients much relieved, knowing that they can get something which they've perceived to work for them.

The whole area of risk, benefit and now cost, has been given a new dimension for us by having to consider another aspect of our clinical practice, which is caring for populations. In formulating clinical policy, one is not only faced with individual counselling, for example with the parents of a child dealing with the benefits of whooping cough vaccination, but also with the population as a whole. That can be extended to many conditions, and a good illustration is the results of the MRC trial which have been invaluable in helping us to make decisions, not only about the individual patient but also about what the policy of the practice as a whole should be with the economic implications for the taxpayer.

This dimension to care is taking those of us in general practice into the question of quality and how it is assessed. The most obvious indicators of outcome relating to money and death are eminently measurable, whereas others are not. The measurement of disability in some conditions, for example in asthmatics, is easier than in the elderly. As doctors we are having to think afresh about how we generally negotiate with patients about their input and perceptions of what quality actually means. Friendliness, kindliness, accessibility and availability are dimensions which are not often on the doctor's agenda, or if they are they have quite a different priority. I am personally sceptical that we will ever be able to compute these neatly into some form of health index, but at least the aim is worth striving for.

The incorporation of the principles of quality assessment into everyday clinical practice stems from the fact tht we are in the business as doctors, and in particular, as general practitioners, of making decisions on the basis of relatively imperfect information. We have to weigh these up for individual people and for the community and come to a conclusion. It implies that we have to overhaul our thinking about management, and we are, therefore, going right outside our consulting rooms to see what principles can be brought from industry to bear on the clinical decision making process, the assessment of benefit and risks. Inevitably, with that, has to go an overhaul and a radical improvement of the database currently available to practices, and which ultimately should lead to a completion of the feedback cycle. We, the clinicians, are at the sharp end and in a position best to observe what the effects of particular drugs are at any particular time.

4.4 Risk-benefit decisions in patient care

Professor D.W. Vere

Various authors have discussed risk-benefit decisions in relation to their predictive aspect for patient care[1-3]. However, they are not always discussing the same thing, some being concerned most with averaged risks and benefits and others with their impact on individuals. Thus it would appear that there is very little sound information available to help a physician when trying to reach a risk-benefit decision on behalf of, or with, an individual patient.

(1) *'Risk' is not usually a simple function of 'benefit', although there may be exceptions*
In using a drug with a narrow therapeutic index, one may try higher doses to gain benefit with the result that risk is likely to increase. However, with many adversities related to drugs, the type B adverse reaction, the bizarre idiosyncratic reaction, is the one that is really feared, however rare it may be. This is in no way related to the benefit that may be obtained from the therapy. Also, as others have pointed out, the benefit depends enormously upon the clinical context. Patients who value a drug's apparent benefit highly are often willing to accept higher unpredictable risks from it.

(2) *The basis of risk resides within the patient as well as in the medicine: it is interactive and may be obscure*
This is one reason why 'no fault' liability makes sense as opposed to 'strict' liability. For example, suppose a patient taking a monoamine oxidase (MAO) inhibitor eats some preserved fish and as a result has severe hypertension and a stroke. If the doctor called out to see that patient then gives pethidine for the pain in his head, his blood pressure falls dangerously. Who would this patient sue, the manufacturer of the MAO inhibitor, the

147

manufacturer of the fish, the manufacturer of the pethidine or the doctor who gave him the pethidine? Most people will instinctively blame the MAO inhibitor as the predisposing factor. But is this sensible? Take the example of a girl who has undetected anti-thrombin 3 deficiency and takes the contraceptive pill. Who is responsible for the adverse effects which may follow? There is no clear-cut logic in this situation, and one has to accept that a considerable part of the risk resides within the patient.

(3) *Most patients do not understand risk; they model it as 'odds' or 'chance' and form emotional preferences towards it*
Although the number of patients who understand risk is increasing in our society, many do not. Some model it as odds simply because they are race-goers, so they feel they know what odds mean. Interestingly enough, I don't think they always do. They may also think about 'chance' or 'fate'. There is a very large Bengali population in the East End of London who will accept the most unbelievable adversities as fate, quite imperturbably in contrast to their British neighbours. So there are emotionally driven preferences, and 'health belief models' are enormously important. If the symptoms of an intercurrent viral infection are believed by the patient to be due to the drug they are taking, then that drug may have to be changed, however reasonably you may analyse the matter with them.

(4) *Problem No. 3 is asymmetric: anticipated risk is not equal to experienced risk*
Generally people become unhappy after experiencing an adverse effect. However, it needn't necessarily be that way. I have known patients who have been extremely anxious about an adverse effect of which they have been warned, but when in fact something happens they find it to be not nearly as bad as they had expected. People have health belief models, they have emotive prejudices usually based upon a linkage with some very frightening experience earlier in their lives or something they have read which has disturbed them. One cannot anticipate that but can only try to cope with it when it occurs.

(5) *Risk of the unchecked disease may or may not be known*
When you are about to treat a patient, you never know what will happen if they are left untreated. Sometimes this phenomenon reaches extreme levels. I remember the arguments about razoxane as a treatment for psoriatic arthropathy. When we were shown pictures of the sufferers, we came to realize that it was only the people who suffered from the extreme forms of the

disease, or those near to them, who really understood what a malignant process this was. In fact it could be worse than the cancer risk from which regulatory authorities had sought to save those patients. In the risk–benefit decisions one has to be very close to an afflicted group to know how it may affect them, how they see the problem, the physical and psychological difficulties and also such things as social stigma associated with their particular illness.

(6) *Risk of loss of treatment efficacy is unknown*
Until very recently, not much was known about the mechanisms of tolerance, tachyphylaxis or failure of treatment. We have all been aware of patients who started off with a very effective therapy, then gradually efficacy was lost. This has been noticed recently with several anti-hypertensive drugs. Good control occurs in some patients over the first 8 months but on continuing, even flexibly with changing dosage, control is lost. We do not know why this happens in one patient but not in the next whose control remains highly effective, although scientific work is beginning to show some potential reasons for this[4].

(7) *Statistical versus individual risk: asymmetric 'before' and 'after' the adverse event*
The asymmetry of risk appreciation is noticeable among those who suffer from drug adversities. It is a very different matter to feel ' I *might* be the one in 10 000' to feel 'I *am* the one in 10 000'.

(8) *Risk varies as disease evolves*
A good example of this is rubella, where people formed views about abortion policy in relation to epidemics. When they put the Policy into effect they found that in some epidemics the incidence of congenital malformation in the aborted foetuses was far lower than they had anticipated. This is not the only disease that varies in severity; the ischaemic heart disease of today is not the same condition that I encountered as a medical student.

(9) *Drug patent 'lives' are now so short that the risk profiles may never become known, especially for less frequent disorders*
As drug sophistication increases the development time goes up, and the effective patent life of a drug in the market becomes shorter and shorter. The 'experience window' becomes smaller, and less is known about that treatment in the field at the time when it comes to be withdrawn.

I think enough has been said today about patients' attitudes to risk. The paper by Barbara McNeil and colleagues in 1978[4] was very revealing about why some patients chose radiotherapy rather than surgery; this was due to the greater immediate risk of death associated with surgery. Immediate survival seemed more prominent in their eyes than the problem of distant survival.

Enough has already been said with regard to the question of the 'non-specificity' of apparent adverse reactions: a symptom may be common to spontaneous disease and to an adverse drug effect. An enormous amount of new information came from studies like that of Bulpitt, Dollery and Carne[5], in which the changes in symptoms of hypertensive patients on referral to hospital were studied comparatively.

Are there any treatments where the scientific knowledge base is becoming sufficiently strong to help in individual decisions in depth? There seem to be very few. One which is changing my clinical practice is the growing knowledge about digoxin. The work of Ford *et al.*[3] on receptor numbers helps me to begin to understand tachyphylaxis in relation to digoxin. There is also Johnston and McDevitt's work[6] on the withdrawal of digoxin from patients with sinus rhythm and heart failure, and the remarkable difficulties for treatment decisions that it revealed. We start a treatment, it works well and we continue with it. Seldom do we know what will happen if it is stopped. In those situations where treatments have been stopped often surprisingly few patients needed to return to the treatment. Yet some undoubtedly did, and this fact poses an enormous problem in risk–benefit analysis for the individual patient.

Good medicine has to be an iterative process. There has to be the opportunity to observe treatment after it has begun, for change in the face of new evidence and experiment for trial and error. There is much bad medicine in the sense that doctors do not follow-up patients at sensitive times. The opportunity to vary the course is therefore missed, and the opportunity to gain the best out of the treatment is lost. Even that is no help with sudden idiosyncratic reactions, although good iterative medicine does avert numerous ill-responses which develop gradually. Lastly, clinical pharmacological research tends to reveal the safest, average pathway to pursue for rational drug use. This minimizes risk, but for the individual one must always be prepared to vary the treatment if it seems right to do so. Some attitudes of hard science fundamentalism, whether among doctors or in professions ancillary to medicine and amongst regulators, are very worrying. Some people seem unable to believe that a drug used at an aberrant dose for an unlicensed indication in a rather expensive way has actually helped a patient.

References

1.   Brimblecombe, R.W. and Dayan, A.D. (1985). Preclinical toxicity testing. In Burley, D.M. and Binns, T.B. (eds.) *Pharmaceutical Medicine,* p.18 (London: Arnold)

2. Teeling-Smith, G. (1983). In Teeling-Smith, G. (ed.). *Measuring the Social Benefits of Medicine.* pp. 163–6 (London: Office of Health Economics.)

3. Ford, A.R., Aronson, J.K., Grahame-Smith, D.G. and Carver, J.G. (1979). The acute changes seen in cardiac glycoside receptor sites during the early phases of digoxin therapy are not found during chronic therapy. *Br. J. Clin. Pharmacol.,* **8**, 135–42

4. McNeil, Barbara, J., Weidselbaum, R. and Pauker, S.G. (1978). Fallacy of the five year survival in lung cancer. *N. Engl. J. Med.,* **299**, 1397–401.

5. Bulpitt, C.J., Dollery, C.T. and Carne, S. (1976). Change in symptoms of hypertensive patients after referral to hospital clinics. *Br. Heart J.,* **38**, 121–8

6. Johnston, G.C. and McDevitt, D.G. (1979). Is maintenance digoxin necessary in patients with sinus rhythm? *Lancet,* **1**, 567–70

4.4 Risk-benefit decisions in patient care

Discussant: Dame E. Ackroyd

The opportunity to discuss frankly the problems in risk–benefit decisions in patient care is encouraging and illuminating. However, all that has been said, very clearly indicates how difficult it is to get it right. We all recognize that most patients do survive to a reasonably old age although some, of course, are in discomfort. This introduces the issue about how the patient with a painful condition sees the costs and benefits. It does not do justice to medical treatment to denigrate it to the extent of thinking that it is a waste of time because people are not deriving any benefit from it. At large, people at the very worst survive their medical treatment.

Speaking on behalf of patients, I do resent the assumption that we are irrational or illogical just because we do not follow a doctor's line of thought. The decisions which we want to make are rational in the light of our social, family or cultural background. Regarding the patient's assessment of this, many are very aware of risk because of their gambling experiences. People do make an assessment of risk. People, increasingly and instinctively in a sense, recognize that in medicine, as in all other things in life, there is some risk attached.

I would like to mention Mrs S. although she was a surgical rather than a pharmaceutical disaster. She had an operation on her shoulder and as a result was permanently disabled. She had started with a pain in her shoulder which had been rather inconvenient and uncomfortable for a number of years. As the surgeon who performed the operation died before the case came to court, what he had actually told her was not known. It was believed he had told her of the risk, but he had not discussed with her the 1% risk which was in fact the one which disabled her. The interesting thing is that Mrs S. says that had she known it was a 1% risk, she would not have had the operation. Quite honestly I am doubtful about that as I believe that most people would accept a 1 in 100 chance, whereas I think they would be dubious about 1 in 20. They would certainly accept 1 in 1000 and when you get above 1000 it is beyond most people's capability to visualize.

Returning to who should take the decision or help the patient to take the decision, of course it is the doctor. Patients do put their doctors on pedestals and it is because they are different. An analogy can be drawn to a plumber, who I expect to have superior knowledge to mine. I do not expect to tell him how to mend the drains, but I expect him to use his knowledge. In the case of the doctor, I have paid for this knowledge. I expect him to have the knowledge and experience which he deploys on the patient's behalf. He should, however, share that knowledge with the patient by explaining the issues, recommending a course of action but also drawing attention to the risks associated with it.

Risk–Benefit Decisions

Discussant: Professor Sir A. Goldberg

Generally, it has been said that the public, on the whole, are not risk illiterate. In my own experience as a doctor for almost 40 years, there have been great changes in the appreciation by the public of the area of drug safety. Drug safety is, in a way, a 'fashion'. It may have been a fashion in the past, with the various perturbations of Digitalis, '606', chloroform, Thalidomide etc., but I believe it is now here to stay. If anything the appreciation of drug safety, particularly by the community, will become greater and greater.

An interesting comment made by John Urquhart concerned the age of perception of risk. I think it is very important that children be taught this. Various teaching programmes of health education in schools have been carried out by Health Education Groups. One in Manchester was very interesting because they had cartoons in which drug safety was brought out for 10–12-year-olds quite well, with questions such as, 'Does this drug do you any good? Is it bad for you?'. This area of drug safety is very important, and it could also be of enormous help to compliance by patients in the long run.

The main points and problems of making a judgement regarding product licensing and licence changes have already been made. Although it can be very difficult it has to be done. Griffin and Diggle analysed the reasons product licences were not given an acceptance on the first occasion over a 10-year period. The primary cause was in fact safety, the second was quality and last was efficacy. That is interesting, but on the whole we have to make a judgement on what, in retrospect, may look like inadequate evidence. Indeed, Sherrington summed it up many years ago when he said that 'science could nobly wait for an answer, but common sense, pressed for time, must act on acceptance'. The record, however, clearly shows that 'safety' has been, as it will always be, a dominant consideration.

Finally, the dialogue and discussions today on the benefit–risk ratio will

155

filter out to the general practitioner. This whole area of discussion of the benefit–risk ratio is becoming more omnipresent in the general medical community. In talking to general practitioners in various parts of the country, this is quite an accepted and common practice. Glasgow patients are in many ways sophisticated and in other ways are unsophisticated, yet one finds that they appreciate that it is important at times not to take any medication at all. In addition, they are becoming more aware of the problems of drug safety.

Risk-Benefit Decisions

Discussion (Chairman: Professor R. Hurley)

DR FITZGERALD: I would like to raise some points with Professor Vere as I think the example of razoxine, with which I was particularly involved, raises some very interesting and general principles. This drug was not approved for the indication of psoriasis. It was found to be associated with a certain incidence of leukaemia (there was no denominator, of course) and we wrote to all the dermatologists who were using it. As a result, a large number of patients were withdrawn from razoxine and several died from a rapid rebound with tremendous exfoliation. It was almost impossible to get over to very intelligent consultant dermatologists that it was not a ban on the use of the drug but a major change in the risk–benefit ratio which they had to discuss with their patients, indicating that the real risk was not known. This is a recent event and I am certain that there is a large number of patients whose quality of life has now dramatically deteriorated because of the information the dermatologists received. I realize that it is a very ambiguous position because it wasn't approved by the licensing authority for this particular indication. But it is a real life situation, and for me highlighted very clearly the large difficulties of trying to explain, even to people who have very considerable experience of clinical medicine, a change in the risk–benefit ratio.

DR CAVALLA: I think that Dame Elizabeth mentioned that patients are not irrational; but I did make the statement that the general public is risk illiterate. I think Desmond supports that in effect by saying that, even to a skilled population, it is very difficult to put the facts over in such a way that the illiteracy is removed. What I see around me at the moment is not very consoling. On the one hand there is an almost determined attempt by the media to dissociate sense and sensibility from the perception of risk; they glory in trivial risks, while in most cases they ignore the larger risks. In the case of the medical scene in general, there are consumer activists who have issues at hand which make it difficult for them to see risk in any sensible terms. There are also politicians who will see the whole question of risk as being necessary for their further benefit as politicians. I think we, as specialists, as medical and physical scientists have a responsibility to put this

157

risk element into perspective as firmly and as frankly as we can, in a manner which as many people as possible can understand. Only by so doing are we going to achieve a sensible resolution of this problem. One speaker referred to the tragedy of Seveso and no doubt many people in this room think it was a tragedy. I assure you it was not; no-one died there, and very few people were rendered ill as a result. On the other hand, it is believed, as a result of the depravations of the media, that Seveso was a tragedy and that is just one example of what I am trying to say.

PROFESSOR DOLLERY: I think that although the discussions we have had today have been very good, they have mostly been skilful apologies for the status quo. Everyone wants the public to be more informed, more aware and to participate in decisions. Yet we operate a very closed system and I would suggest that if we seriously want to achieve those objectives we might consider changing the way we do things. I would, therefore, like to make some suggestions.

(1)   Allow anyone with a home computer to access the CSM database on the yellow cards, so that there would be no mystery about what was and was not contained in the records.

(2)   The submissions to the CSM when a drug is licensed should be made available to everyone either immediately, or perhaps after a delay of 3 years to protect the commercial interests. There is very little in the submissions that after 3 years would be of any commercial value to anybody. I think people are concerned that we are all concealing something, which to some extent we are. Perhaps if people knew that problems were creeping up all the time they wouldn't become alarmed when one comes out of the woodwork.

(3)   One of the things that worries me about present policy in assessing benefit–risk is that it is so square. The CSM will decide either to do nothing or to withdraw a drug, very often. I think that is a questionable policy. For example, when a drug is withdrawn it would often be more sensible to recommend that no new patients start the drug, as a withdrawal decision can create havoc for people already on a drug.

(4)   It would be helpful if the industry could take a much more positive aspect to safety. It should be more willing to use their considerable powers of persuasion to the professions through their detail force and advertisements to also tell people when not to use drugs. They do teach people something about contra-indications, but they don't actively go out and explain situations when a drug should not be used. As a consequence drugs are often used in instances where they should not be. I have read the files on osmosin and benoxaprofen from the manufacturers and there is no doubt that a number of the most severe adverse reactions occurred when the drug was being used inappropriately, or was continued when patients were suffering from clinical features which should have rung a strong warning bell.

I think, therefore, that if we would become less complacent and change the system it would be for the better.

PROFESSOR GOLDBERG: Speaking personally, I think if one had to take a vote of members of the CSM, the great majority of them would want to be as open as they possibly could. There are, however, legal problems relating to industry which are mitigating in this particular area. Our aim is increasingly to try and communicate as much as possible about adverse reactions and the benefit-risk ratio. Regarding the withdrawal of licences, I think Colin is right in that there are problems ensuing from the abrupt withdrawal of particular drugs. However, we do appreciate the problems Colin has enunciated, and we have tried to predict and prevent these. In the five and a half years I have been with the CSM there have been changes in the way we work, and there will be further changes in the next five.

DR URQUHART: In relation to what Professor Dollery said, there is a model of this in the United States. It came up after the cyclamate/saccharin controversy, which threw the food industry into a terrible turmoil. They set up the 'Foods Safety Council' which endeavoured to produce an outline for food additive safety testing. Everyone who could conceivably be interested was brought into the discussion, and a report was produced which has since served as a guideline for food safety evaluation. In the process everyone, including the media, became so bored with the subject that it all blew over. What was a confusing arena in 1973 had completely quietened down by 1976. That could historically be regarded as a model for what could be done in the pharmaceutical industry.

PROFESSOR RAWLINS: I agree in principle with what Colin has suggested, but it would of course require a repeal of Section 118 of the Medicines Act, with a few other changes. However, that only solves the problem of public acceptance; it does not solve the problem of how to assess risk and benefit. At least part of the trouble is the lack of good data from which to base the assessment, and unless that is corrected I don't think we will be able to correct the rest.

PROFESSOR WALKER: We have had a very interesting discussion this afternoon and have seen some of the deficiencies in the data on which we make these benefit–risk decisions. However, so far there have been no recommendations as to how we might improve the situation in the future, and, therefore, be in a better position to make risk–benefit decisions at the various stages in the development of a new drug.

PROFESSOR INMAN: I believe that we cannot progress until people sit down and decide what risks are acceptable and reach a consensus view for individual types of disease. As John Griffin pointed out, if you need 46000 patients to identify a 1 in 10000 risk, this may be important for one disease but not for another.

DR GRIFFIN: I would like to endorse not only what Bill has said, but also the fact that we will have to go to post-marketing surveillance. The cohort size, which is limiting, is going to determine what risks will be acceptable in the future. We will be limited by the practicality of what can be done with PMS.

In order to assess 'risk' we have to be quite sure that we distinguish 'real risk' from 'perceived risk'. There can be a marked difference between impression and reality. To assess 'risk' associated with any medical treatment there have to be a number of factors known with some degree of accuracy.

(1) *The detection of side-effects*

Because serious adverse reactions are usually rare they are difficult to detect. If the incidence of serious ADR were 1:10 000 then the number of reports expected in a series of 100 patients is only 0.01. Clearly the probability of detecting any is remotely small. If the number of patients studied is increased to 1000 the probability is only 10%, if to 10 000 it becomes 63%, still insufficiently high. To increase the probability of detecting any ADR at all with a probability of 99% it would be necessary to study about 46 000 patients. Let us suppose that a drug adversely affected one patient among every 10 000 treated: there would be only 1% chance of encountering a single case in a 100-patient trial. In 100 similar trials, we might easily dismiss one case as a chance event.

(2) *The incidence of side-effects may vary*

Any particular treatment may produce a range of side-effects, each with varying incidence depending on circumstances, e.g. benoxaprofen produced photosensitivity reactions with an incidence varying between 10–30 per 100 patients treated. This, however, varied with intensity of sunlight, and consequently showed a geographical distribution. Hepatorenal syndrome occurred with an incidence of about 1 in 6–8000, but the risk increased with duration of exposure.

The incidence of vincristine neuropathy is greater in patients with Hodgkins' lymphoma than in patients with non-Hodgkins' lymphoma or leukaemia at comparable dose levels (Watkins and Griffin, 1978).

Pulmonary adverse reactions to nitrofurantoin occur at greater frequency in Sweden than in the UK, with Holland in an intermediate position. Conversely, nitrofurantoin neuropathy occurs more frequently in the UK than in Sweden (Griffin and Penn, 1980). Side-effects may be commoner in the elderly or in children.

(3) *Severity of side-effects*

Certain side-effects may be common but trivial, others may be rarer but severe. Even having detected the occurrence of a side-effect the severity and its sequelae may differ when caused by different therapeutic agents, e.g. halothane jaundice has a high mortality, erythromycin jaundice a very low one. The severity of side-effects can only be determined when a considerable series has been built up.

(4) *Risk of side-effects of long latency*

It is absolutely clear that assessment of risk based on clinical data, even involving several thousand patients as is now the case with most new chemical entities (NCEs), is a pretty crude assessment. The risk of side-effects of long latency, e.g. teratogenicity, carcinogenicity, etc. is largely a judgement based on extrapolation from animal toxicity data.

(5) *Balancing the risk of disease versus risk of treatment*
The risk of disease in terms of incidence and outcome in terms of mortality and morbidity are seldom formally assessed in current therapeutics. We should re-examine this practice, particularly where we are considering risk in terms of prophylaxis as opposed to treatment of individual sick patients.

(6) *Perception of risk change*
Clearly we have to accept that at the time of granting marketing approval of a New Chemical Entity (NCE) we are making arbitrary judgements based on, of necessity, incomplete data. When we make, so called, risk–benefit judgements before allowing an NCE onto the market there is a tendency for these judgements to be more restrictive if they are taken in temporal proximity to an earlier drug-related disaster. In other words, the goal posts move perceptibly in the wake of events such as practolol and benoxaprofen, but more insidiously in the wake of more minor events. However, the escalation in demands for more clinical data is really too small to increase the predictive value of judgements, but is sufficient to increase cost in both financial terms and erosion of patent life.

(7) *Post-marketing surveillance (PMS)*
Clearly the number of patients exposed to enable a proper assessment of incidence and severity of potential adverse reactions to an NCE is far greater than could be demanded in clinical trials. It must, therefore, be accepted that all NCEs will require PMS studies. Having made this step it should be possible to make some assessment as to what the acceptable incidence of side-effects for different therapeutic groups would be, bearing in mind the risks from the disease and comparable levels of risk from other available treatments for the disease (for rare diseases, e.g. Wilson's disease, such PMS procedures may be inappropriate).
    Once the broad magnitude of the PMS study that should be required for each therapeutic class has been laid down, and the problem looked at in cold terms it should become apparent that many of the demands made for pre-marketing clinical evaluation would be more appropriately met in the PMS phase.

References

1. Watkins, S.M. and Griffin, J.P. (1978). High incidence of vincristine-induced neuropathy in lymphomas. *Br. Med. J.,* **1**, 1610–12
2. Griffin, J.P. and Penn, R.G. (1980). Adverse reactions to nitrofurantoin in UK, Sweden and Holland. *Br. Med. J.,* **248**, 1440–

Index